PHILOSOPHIC WHIGS

THE WELLCOME INSTITUTE SERIES IN THE HISTORY OF MEDICINE

Edited by W.F. Bynum and Roy Porter
The Wellcome Institute

Florence Nightingale and the Nursing Legacy
Monica Baly

Vivisection in Historical Perspective
Nicholas A. Rupke

Abortion in England, 1900–1967
Barbara Brookes

The Hospital in History
Lindsay Granshaw and Roy Porter

The Charitable Imperative
Colin Jones

Medicine at the Courts of Europe, 1500–1837
Vivian Nutton

Mad Tales from the Raj
Waltraud Ernst

British Medicine in an Age of Reform
Roger French and Andrew Wear

Doctor of Society
Roy Porter

Medical Journals and Medical Knowledge
W.F. Bynum, Stephen Lock and Roy Porter

Medical Theory, Surgical Practice
Christopher Lawrence

The Popularization of Medicine, 1650–1860
Roy Porter

Women and Children First
Valerie Fildes, Lara Marks and Hilary Marland

Psychiatry for the Rich
Charlotte MacKenzie

Literature and Medicine during the Eighteenth Century
Marie Mulvey Roberts and Roy Porter

The Art of Midwifery
Hilary Marland

Medicine and the Reformation
Ole Peter Grell and Andrew Cunningham

Sophia Jex-Blake
Shirley Roberts

PHILOSOPHIC WHIGS

Medicine, Science and Citizenship in Edinburgh, 1789–1848

L.S. Jacyna

London and New York

First published 1994
by Routledge
11 New Fetter Lane, London EC4P 4EE

Simultaneously published in the USA and Canada
by Routledge
29 West 35th Street, New York, NY 10001

Typeset in Baskerville by LaserScript, Mitcham, Surrey
Printed and bound in Great Britain by
Biddles Ltd, Guildford and King's Lynn

British Library Cataloguing in Publication Data
A catalogue record for this book is available from the British Library.

Library of Congress Cataloging in Publication Data
Jacyna, L.S.
Philosophic whigs: medicine, science, and citizenship in Edinburgh, 1789–1848/L.S. Jacyna.
p. cm. – (The Wellcome Institute series in the History of Medicine)
Includes bibliographical references and index.
1. Medicine – Scotland – Edinburgh – History – 18th century.
2. Medicine – Scotland – Edinburgh – History – 19th century.
3. University of Edinburgh. Faculty of Medicine – History – 18th century. 4. University of Edinburgh. Faculty of Medicine – History – 19th century. 5. Medicine – Political aspects – Scotland – Edinburgh – History – 18th century.
6. Medicine – Political aspects – Scotland – Edinburgh – History – 19th century. 7. Physicians – Scotland – Edinburgh – Biography. 8. Thomson family. I. Title. II. Series.
[DNLM: 1. History of Medicine, 19th Cent. – Scotland.
2. Physicians – Scotland – biography. 3. Schools, Medical – History – Scotland. 4. Politics – Scotland. WZ 70 FS2 J2h 1994]
R497.E34J33 1994
610′.9413′409034 – dc20
DNLM/DLC
for Library of Congress 93-29944
ISBN 0-415-03614-3

Contents

Abbreviations

BL MS	British Library Manuscripts Department
ECA	Edinburgh City Archives
EUL MS	Edinburgh University Library Special Collections
GUL MS	Glasgow University Library Special Collections
LSE	London School of Economics
NLS	National Library of Scotland, Edinburgh
PRO	Public Records Office, Kew
RCPE	Royal College of Physicians of Edinburgh
RCSE	Royal College of Surgeons of Edinburgh
SRO	Scottish Records Office, Edinburgh
WIHM	Wellcome Institute for the History of Medicine, London

Introduction

In 1789 John Thomson left Glasgow to continue his medical studies in Edinburgh. In 1848 his youngest son Allen resigned the post he held in the Edinburgh medical faculty to become Professor of Anatomy in Glasgow. In the intervening half century members of the Thomson family occupied a total of four chairs in Edinburgh; evolved new forms of pedagogy; practised surgery and medicine; and took an active part in the cultural life and politics of the city.

This book is primarily an account of the Thomson family's Edinburgh career. As such it helps to fill a lacuna in our understanding of the Edinburgh medical school. Conventionally historians have focussed their attention upon the eighteenth-century 'Golden Age' of Edinburgh medicine which is supposed to have ended around 1789 with the retirement of William Cullen. The fascination of this earlier period is easily understood. It coincides with the efflorescence of the Scottish Enlightenment; this was the Edinburgh of Adam Smith and David Hume as well as of Cullen and of Joseph Black. Among the most stimulating studies of this period are those which emphasize the intimate relations between medicine and other forms of intellectual endeavour.[1]

By contrast, the turn of the nineteenth century appears as a period of decline for the medical school. The great men had passed away to be replaced by unworthy successors. This image of decline was well defined even in the early decades of the nineteenth century: in 1825 an English visitor to the northern Athens noted that, with minor exceptions,

> I did not hear that any of the Athenian professors have put in a single claim for immortality. Even in her anatomical school, that upon which she rested her fame the longest and the most securely, the recent falling off has been great; and of all those who now shine in the lists of her *senatus* there is none able to hold the book for Gregory, or the scalpel for old Monro, or light the furnace for Black.[2]

In the view of this author the causes of the decline were clear: they were the fruit of faction and of the injudicious distribution of patronage that flowed from it. More recent commentators have tended to confirm this diagnosis of the sources of the Edinburgh medical school's malaise at the turn of the nineteenth century.[3]

Various objections might be raised to this admittedly satisfying narrative of glory followed by corruption and decline. Recent studies of the Brunonian controversies in the 1780s have shown the possibility of strife even in the age of gold.[4] Nor was the distribution of university patronage in the eighteenth century immune to the demands of faction. It is none the less undeniable that the school of medicine was more riven by conflict after 1790 than before. This was, however, a reflection of the tendency of Edinburgh society as a whole.

University histories are prone to what may be called the 'green field' syndrome – a tendency to view these institutions as ivory towers devoted to the pursuit of eternal values and detached from the more mundane concerns of their environment. Even as sophisticated a study as Lisa Rosner's recent history of the medical school at the turn of the nineteenth century gives little idea of the dependence of academic institutions upon a larger social context.[5] This pastoral perspective is particularly ill-adapted to the history of Edinburgh University. Its title as the 'Town's College' was no mere form of words but a reflection of the university's complete integration into the political economy of the city. In Thomas Bender's words, Edinburgh University was 'so indeterminate in its structure and reach that university and city are nearly assimilated into each other'.[6] By the 1790s, moreover, the Edinburgh polity had lost much of its former independence; improved communications facilitated the subordination of local to national interests.

From the 1780s the political nation experienced growing conflict between those who wished to preserve the existing constitution and those who demanded some measure of reform. In Scotland this struggle centred upon the issues of parliamentary representation and burgh government. The questions were interrelated because the Town Councils elected the members of parliament for Scottish cities. The councils were themselves unelected self-perpetuating bodies subservient to the will of the party in power and notoriously corrupt.[7]

The Tory guardians of this system were both ruthless in the defence of their privileges and shameless in exploiting its potentials for furthering their own interests as well as those of family and friends. In Mudie's words, 'The Athenian Tories are perhaps the most place-devoted race in the British dominions. Office is their god.'[8] Academic offices formed part of this system of patronage. Among its other prerogatives, the Town Council of Edinburgh was the patron of the university: most chairs were in its gift and were reserved for those who professed acceptable opinions or who were able to offer some *quid pro quo.* An analyst of the decline of the medical faculty complained in 1834 that 'political intrigue, base jobbing, and even open mercantile barter' had all too often triumphed in academic appointments.[9] Tories were no less aware of the punitive possibilities of a monopoly of patronage; they enforced their authority by 'letting people feel that they have the dispensing of rewards; by standing between a candidate and an office for which he is qualified, or by something of a similar kind'.[10]

The Revolution in France set these conflicts into sharper relief. While the advocates of reform welcomed at least the early stages of the Revolution as an augury of a more general instauration, reactionaries saw the overthrow of the *ancien régime* as confirmation of the dangers of all innovation. After the events of 1792–3, anyone who still called for domestic reform ran the risk of being branded not merely foolish but as a traitor to his country and a menace to the social order. The history of Edinburgh was thus entwined with the course of events on the Continent. A concrete reminder of the lessons to be drawn from the constitutional experiment in France was supplied by the presence of the Comte d'Artois who, after his brother's execution, took up quarters in Holyrood Palace along with a train of French nobles.

John Thomson came to Edinburgh a few months after the Estates General convened. His subsequent fortunes showed with exceptional clarity how a medical career could be structured by this political environment. Indeed, from the outset Thomson elected to be a political as well as a professional actor upon the Edinburgh stage; he aspired to be a citizen as well as a surgeon. While still a student, he ostentatiously aligned himself with the Whig opponents of the prevalent regime and made public his sympathies for the first proceedings of the French Revolution.

While he later tempered his enthusiasm for the latter event, Thomson never abandoned his Whig principles; he therefore invited the opprobrium and ostracism the establishment reserved for its opponents. His fellow medical student and political confrère John Allen faced the same persecution. But while Allen left Edinburgh and abandoned medicine, Thomson persevered in his goal of establishing himself as medical practitioner and teacher in Edinburgh; and, to a remarkable degree, he triumphed over his enemies. Much of the fascination of his career lies in the means he employed to circumvent the obstacles placed before him.

The state of the medical school at the turn of the nineteenth century offered opportunities as well as pitfalls. The decline of the medical faculty provided a vacuum for enterprising extramural teachers to fill. The Royal College of Surgeons of Edinburgh constituted an alternative focus to the university medical school – one which, moreover, displayed a greater degree of political independence. The College traced its antecedents to the Surgeons and Barbers Corporation erected in 1505. In 1657 the surgeons had been united with the city's apothecaries and from this date set aside their business as barbers. While not the oldest of the Edinburgh trades, the Corporation of Surgeons was the senior city guild and took precedence on ceremonial occasions. The surgeons were thus an integral part of the traditional establishment of the city; their Deacon was, for instance, ex officio a member of the Town Council.[11] During the last quarter of the eighteenth century, however, the surgeons began to aspire to a new identity: they sought to transform a local trade guild into an educational and licensing body with a national ambit. They wished, in short, to cease to be artisans and to become gentlemen professing a liberal science. Symbolic of these ambitions was the new charter they obtained in 1778 that named them 'The Royal College of Surgeons of the City of Edinburgh'.[12] John Thomson made adroit use of the surgeons' aspirations to form an alternative centre of medical education in Edinburgh to further his own aspirations.

Politics were given added acerbity by the fact that the nation was at war and at times menaced by invasion. But the same circumstance also generated a resource for an enterprising medical teacher to exploit. In the course of the revolutionary and Napoleonic wars Edinburgh underwent an unpredented militarization: in 1803 there were some 10,000 soldiers billeted in and around the city. To accommodate these troops, new barracks were erected on the west side of the castle and a cavalry depot built at Piershill.[13] The military was, in short, a major presence and power in Edinburgh during these years; John Thomson demonstrated that they could also be turned into a patron.

For twenty years he cultivated the army authorities and derived numerous benefits from the relationship; above all, it was as a professor of military surgery that he first gained entry to the university. Although these links became less important later in Thomson's career, he continued to draw half pay as a staff surgeon until his death.[14] He seems, moreover, to have taken seriously his military persona; in 1822 Thomson attended George IV's levee in Edinburgh '*en militaire*'.[15]

In pursuit of his goals Thomson made use of the services of various individuals. His elder son William was, in particular, a faithful instrument. An 'adopted' son such as Robert Carswell or John William Turner could also be drawn into the family enterprise when they had serviceable talents to offer. An important aspect of this study is the way in which Thomson's teaching firm evolved new doctrines and pedagogic technologies in its efforts to establish a niche within the Edinburgh market for medical education. Pathological anatomy, auscultation and microscopy were among the tools that were adapted to their professional ends. Foreign medical schools were intensively explored and exploited to provide new pedagogic resources. While the Faculty of Medicine may have declined in the early nineteenth century, this was not a period of stagnation in medical education: on the contrary, innovation was a by-product of the competitive demands placed upon extramural teachers.

The chronicle of the Thomson family also illustrates the emergence of new medical identities in the course of the early nineteenth century. John Thomson combined the roles of teacher and practitioner to the end of his career; his elder son did likewise. Carswell, however, progressively emancipated himself from his preceptor's demands and became a pure pathologist. Allen Thomson, the youngest member of the family firm, also eschewed practice for pedagogy and the pursuit of medical science; his chosen field was physiology. With the possible exception of Carswell all these professional identities were combined with a pronounced and self-conscious political identity. The Thomsons were not *merely* medical practitioners, teachers and investigators; they saw the pursuit of their various professional avocations as both instrumental to the furtherance of the Whig cause and as the fulfilment of the precepts of a particular concept of citizenship.

Although John Thomson and his immediate affines are the protagonists of this study, it also takes account of other philosophic Whigs. Scottish Whiggery was of a different character to its aristocratic English counterpart. It was more the property of professional men who gave a keen intellectual edge and a greater coherence to the eclectic Whig programme. Above all, Scottish Whigs developed political economy as a 'scientific' foundation for their creed. Their ethos eschewed, however, any form of narrow specialization; they felt it incumbent on them to develop a wide range of literary and scientific interests. Although overtly progressive, they none the less drew upon the ideas and ideals of 'Old' Whiggery in response to the extreme conditions of the 1790s.

I have discussed the career and ideas of Thomson's fellow medical student John Allen at some length. He was a startlingly radical and vigorous thinker for which he paid the price. Allen's lectures on physiology in particular illustrate the systematic links that existed between structures of medical and social discourse. Allen left Edinburgh at an early date and settled in London; ensconced in Holland House he became the chief conduit through which the intellectual resources of Scottish Whiggery became available to the party's metropolitan leadership. Allen continued, moreover, to exert an action at a distance upon his former base; his name recurs throughout this book.

The first chapter attempts the more general task of defining the milieu in which Allen and Thomson sought to establish a civic identity upon their arrival in Edinburgh. It seeks to establish the character of philosophic Whiggism as a response to the environment of repression that prevailed in the city at the turn of the nineteenth century; and, in particular, to show how in this context participation in science could be a political act – an aspect of the *vita activa* not merely of a *vita contemplativa*.

In writing this book I have been able to draw upon the large and excellent literature that now exists on the Scottish Enlightenment and on eighteenth-century British political thought. The current scholarship on nineteenth-century Scotland is less helpful. Anand Chitnis is one of the few to try to trace the transition from the Enlightenment to the Victorian era;[16] in the process he discusses many of the same individuals who figure in the present volume. His treatment is, however, superficial. By confining his problematic to the 'influence' of Scottish ideas on English institutions, he overlooks other more searching questions. There is, in particular, little sense of the role of 'Scottish' ideas and of their proponents in the political struggles of the period. There was no simple process of assimilation of Scottish cultural products during this period; nor were these resources generated in an autonomous sphere of intellectual endeavour. Although Chitnis encompasses medicine, his discussion amounts to little more than a catalogue of the activities of certain Scottish-trained practitioners south of the border.

Philosophic Whigs was not written to vindicate any particular methodological programme. It does, however, exemplify a number of interpretative principles the relevance of which extends beyond the immediate subject matter of this book. The work can be seen as an extended essay on the inescapable presence of the political in the world of nineteenth-century medicine. At its most basic this proposition can be taken to refer to the fact that anyone seeking to make a career in medicine in early nineteenth-century Edinburgh had to be prepared to negotiate a terrain populated by such sentient agents as the university, the medical corporations, and the military. Such beings could be appeased, flattered, accommodated, or challenged; but they could not be ignored. Moreover, the categories of classical political analysis were also present and potent. Whether he was 'Whig' or 'Tory' was a matter of some importance in deciding a medical man's future. Medical patronage was in principle no different from any other of the forms of largesse used to lubricate the wheels of the machine of state.

But the medical estate *was* peculiar in its superintendence over a particular class of cultural production. This study shows how physiological texts could also be imbued with political meaning and adapted to serve political purposes. This is perhaps no longer a startling claim: Adrian Desmond has, for instance, made this proposition central to his account of the lineaments of comparative anatomy in early nineteenth-century London.[17] I believe that it is possible to speak of 'Whig science' in Edinburgh in the period between 1790 and 1830, but only in much more guarded terms that those in which Desmond uses to characterize the 'radical' science that he discerns in contemporary London. In the first place, despite the close personal links and strong group solidarity evinced by the Whig party in Edinburgh during this period, its members were by no means an ideologically homogenous group. The cautious and ornate moderation of Dugald Stewart stood in sharp contrast to the more extreme philosophical stance of some of the younger members of the party. Nor can any single scientific doctrine be identified as peculiarly characteristic of the faction or as expressive of their cosmology and interests. None the less, various of the medical discourses discussed in this book did possess both an expressive significance and an instrumental political value.

To discern the various uses and meanings of medical knowledge, it is necessary to distinguish between different levels and forms of political engagement, while bearing in mind that all such distinctions involve an artificial abstraction from a concrete historical reality. At the level of the 'purely' professional it is useful to conceive of knowledge as a commodity: as something manufactured or bought to be sold at a profit in the medical market-place. In this context there is a necessary confusion between knowledge as proposition and knowledge as performance; to say that John Thomson helped to establish the science of pathological anatomy in Britain is to allude to the fact that he made possible pathological anatomy as a pedagogic option (see chapter 4).

Another level may be discerned in which the purity of professional endeavour becomes somewhat adulterated with the interests of party. Thus Thomson's return to extramural teaching in the 1820s can be understood merely as a professional response to the rebuff that his attempts to obtain a chair for himself in the Faculty of Medicine had suffered. Given the factional nature of the appointments that had been made to the chairs of the theory and practice of medicine, the courses that Thomson and his son offered in these subjects were also statements of political defiance. The content of this teaching, with its lengthy and ostentatious tribute to Dugald Stewart's psychology, reinforced the point. The carefully edited version of Lamarckianism included in the Thomsons' lectures might also be seen as an exemplification of Whig principle because it was both progressive and prudent.

John Allen's case illustrates the consequences of an abandonment of such prudence. He was by far the closest approximation to a 'radical materialist' among the individuals considered in this book. He was, moreover, prepared to make his views known in the public spaces of the Royal Medical Society and in his lectures on physiology in Surgeon's Square (see chapter 2). Allen presented a vision of the animal oeconomy as an autonomous material system that was deeply shocking to the sensibilities of most of his contemporaries. His punishment was ostracism and exile. His actions may be construed as a demonstrative use of medical knowledge designed perhaps to signal independence and defiance of the political establishment but interpreted by the members of that establishment as a challenge to their authority that could not be ignored.

The lectures on physiology that Allen Thomson gave some thirty years later may seem at an opposite pole. Cautious and conventional in his representation of the animal body and of the human mind, the younger Thomson gave few hostages to fortune (see chapter 5). At a deeper level continuities in the concepts of the body articulated by Allen and Thomson are, however, discernible. These represent a more subtle but no less marked instance of how medical knowledge can be imbued with the values, yearnings and mentality of the historical actors who devise and disseminate it.

This volume marks the end of a long immersion in Edinburgh Whiggery. The research on which it is based was made possible by the Wellcome Trust who funded my work in Scotland for a period of four years. It was written in Manchester, and thanks are due to my colleagues, Roger Cooter, Mary Fissell and Steven Sturdy for providing an agreeable and stimulating environment. I am also grateful to Mike Barfoot, Chris Lawrence and Roy Porter for their comments on various drafts of the text. I hope that *Philosophic Whigs* may serve to draw attention to the intellectual richness of nineteenth-century Scottish medicine and to the wealth of material available to the student. Much remains to be done.

1

Philosophic Whiggism

Introduction

Henry Cockburn in the *Memorials of his Time* (1856) provided a famous account of the Whig party in Edinburgh at the turn of the nineteenth century. He represented them as a small embattled group surrounded by powerful and vindictive enemies; the 'real *Whigs*', he declared, were extremely few. 'Self-interest had converted some, and terror more; and the residue, which stood out, consisted of only the stronger-minded men of the party'.[1] Among these men of 'rational opinions' Cockburn was especially concerned with a tight-knit set who first rose to prominence in the 1790s: Henry Brougham, Francis Horner and Francis Jeffrey, were its leading members. These are famous names. They were the moving force behind the establishment of the *Edinburgh Review* in 1802, and they went on to have distinguished political careers.[2] A few professors in the University of Edinburgh, notably Dugald Stewart and John Playfair, acted as their allies and mentors. While 'John Allen and John Thomson, of the medical profession, were active and fearless' in the Whig cause.[3]

Cockburn's characterization of Francis Jeffrey as a 'philosophical Whig' can be extended to the group as a whole.[4] This appellation can be construed in various ways.[5] It might signify a propensity to explore the philosophical foundations of political action – a conviction of the need to return politics to first principles: in Dugald Stewart's words,

> In order to lay a solid foundation for the science of politics, the first step ought to be, to ascertain that form of society which is perfectly agreeable to nature and justice; and what are the principles of legislation necessary for maintaining it'.[6]

But 'philosophic Whiggism' might also imply that in order to be a Whig, one needed also to be a philosopher. Philosophy in this context possessed a very wide denotation; it comprised 'the knowledge of those numerous existents or beings that compose the universe, and of those various events which compose the phenomena of the universe'.[7] On this definition, philosophy encompassed the natural as well as the social world; a philosophic Whig might in consequence be expected to be not only a political but also a natural philosopher.

In Edinburgh during the 1790s this logical possibility became a reality. One of the main foci of the Whig community was a shared interest in natural science. John Allen and John Thomson, the two medical Whigs mentioned by Cockburn, played an important enabling role in these activities: they acted as purveyors of scientific knowledge to an intellectually voracious group of consumers. In this chapter I want to consider the ideological dimension of this interest in the natural sciences; to reconstruct an ethos in which the pursuit of science might be seen as expressive of and integral to a particular form of political commitment.

John Thomson and the lure of chemistry

According to Henry Brougham, John Thomson 'was called by his contemporaries "the most learned of physicians"'. Brougham added that 'the discursive character of his scientific acquirements rendered him valuable to the body of young men in Edinburgh, who, at the beginning of the century, were ambitious of adding physical science to their acquirements in law, politics, and general scholarship'. Thomson served this function chiefly by providing instruction in chemistry, a science which possessed a particular appeal to these young men. He seemed to have made a lasting impression; in 1835 the now Lord Chancellor Brougham visited the elderly and ailing Thomson and the two 'talked over their old chemical recreations as if they were still young students with the world before them'.[8]

John Thomson's early career was a tribute to the genuinely democratic possibilities of the Scottish educational system.[9] Born the son of a Paisley silk weaver and apprenticed to his father's trade at the age of eleven, he rose to be a professor in the University of Edinburgh. The transition is somewhat less startling when the high level of literacy among the Paisley websters is recognized: they were said to possess 'libraries equal to those of ministers and professional men'.[10] This lends credibility to the story that Thomson

> laid the foundation for his future eminence by laborious study while following [his father's occupation]. He had the books he was studying always lying open at the side of his loom, and never lost a moment he could spare in making use of them'.[11]

The handloom weavers of the west of Scotland were also noted throughout the eighteenth century for their activism[12]; it is likely that Thomson was exposed to 'advanced' political views at an early age. Thomson's enemies in later life did not forget his social origins: an anonymous denunciation sent to the War Office in 1817 alleged that 'this man by his political intrigues his violence against Government & democratic Principles raised himself from being a Journey Man weaver . . . to his present situation'.[13]

Having persuaded his father that neither weaving nor the church were suitable careers for him, Thomson spent three years apprenticed to a local surgeon. During the 1788–9 session he attended medical classes in Glasgow where he paid special attention to chemistry. The novel doctrines of Lavoisier were at this time giving 'much interest to the proceedings of a society of young and ardent cultivators of chemical science' to which Thomson attached himself.[14] His time in Glasgow may have made a further contribution to the development of Thomson's politics. The University of Glasgow possessed at this time a reputation as a seminary of Whiggism largely through the influence of John Millar, the Professor of Civil Law. Millar later enjoyed the reputation of 'having formed the minds of many of those who have been distinguished in the political world on the liberal side during the last fifty or sixty years'.[15] There is no evidence that Thomson met Millar during his time in Glasgow; he is known, however, to have engaged shortly afterwards in political activities with Millar's eldest son; and in 1806 Thomson married the third of John Millar's seven daughters.[16]

Thomson came to Edinburgh to continue his medical studies in the auspicious year 1789. He was indentured to a surgeon of the city in whose house he first met John Allen a fellow apprentice. Later Allen and Thomson served together as residents at the Royal Infirmary.[17] Allen's father was a Writer to the Signet and owned a small estate near Edinburgh. But for his father's bankruptcy, Allen would have pursued a career in the law. Medicine was a poor second choice; and Allen never had any real taste for medical practice as opposed to medical science.[18]

Thomson and Allen shared politics as well as a profession. They were involved in the organization of the famous or infamous dinner at the Fortune Tavern to celebrate the fall of the Bastille – 'an event so interesting to mankind as the redemption of twenty-six millions from servitude, an event that promised unexampled happiness to the human race' – in the words of the advertisement for the gathering.[19] Allen also became a member of the Society of the Friends of the People and participated in the British Convention that met in Edinburgh in 1792 to call for parliamentary reform much to the alarm of the authorities.[20]

At the same time both men began to be known among the rising generation of Edinburgh literati as men of science and learning as well as of sound political views. During Thomson's early years in Edinburgh, in addition to his strictly professional studies, 'Chemistry . . . occupied a considerable share of his attention.' The publication in 1800 of an edition of Fourcroy's *Elements of Chemistry* was public testimony to those labours.[21]

Thomson appended copious notes to the edition in which he thanked 'his friend Mr Allen for the Notes on Caloric . . . and for the greater part of the Notes on Animal Substances';[22] the two were clearly working in close collaboration.

By the later 1790s Thomson had thus established a reputation in Edinburgh as an authority on chemistry and particularly on *French* chemistry. This status helps to explain an approach he received late in 1799:

> During that winter the late Earl of Lauderdale came to reside in Edinburgh, and being, with that ardour which characterized him in all his pursuits, very desirous to prosecute the study of chemistry, Mr Thomson was introduced to him as a person qualified to assist him.

Under Lauderdale's patronage, 'a chemical class was formed, consisting chiefly of gentlemen connected with the Parliament House, and which met at Mr Thomson's private residence'.[23]

The allusion to 'gentlemen of the Parliament House' requires some elucidation. No parliament had sat in Edinburgh since the Act of Union of 1707. The buildings in Parliament Square retained, however, their function as the seat of the Court of Session; in the words of a nineteenth-century wag, 'although laws are no longer manufactured, they are now retailed, within [the Parliament House], to all who have cash and courage enough to buy them'.[24] The gentlemen in question were therefore the lawyers for whom the Parliament House was a centre for social intercourse as well as for business.[25]

The audience for Thomson's private chemistry class therefore comprised a group of lawyers gathering under the auspices of a member of the aristocracy. The role of aristocrats as patrons of science in eighteenth-century Britain is sufficiently well known; the collective participation of *lawyers* in scientific activities was, however, a peculiarly Scottish phenomenon. It was an aspect of the unique position occupied by the legal profession in the social, political and cultural life of Scotland in the eighteenth and for much of the nineteenth century. Nowhere was this more the case than in the country's capital. The law, declared an English visitor in 1825,

> is [Edinburgh's] Alpha and her Omega, – the food which she eats, the raiment she puts on, the dwelling-house which she inhabits, the conversation in which she engages, the soul which animates her whole frame, the mind which is discovered in every feature of her countenance, and every attitude of her body.[26]

In the post-Union period a close alliance developed between the legal profession in Edinburgh and the landed classes. Gentry families sent their younger sons to study for the law while successful lawyers invested in land. Often the same individual filled both roles: John Allen's father was both a Writer to the Signet and owned an estate. Lauderdale himself had qualified as an advocate in 1780. The legal profession was by virtue of these links an essential part of the civic leadership of eighteenth-century Scotland.[27] They also exercised a great deal of political power. Scotland had little in the way of central government for most of the eighteenth century; but such executive functions as remained in Edinburgh were discharged by the Law Officers of the Crown.[28] Finally, lawyers aspired to a leading part in the *intellectual* life of the country. Although they may not have been outstanding among the authors of the high Scottish Enlightenment, lawyers were prominent in the clubs and societies dedicated to the assimilation and discussion of the new knowledge.[29] Nor did the legal profession participate in these intellectual pursuits in a spirit of idle dilettantism: they saw such engagement with developments in the arts and sciences as integral to their role as the defenders of Scottish liberties, guardians of the nation's virtue, and trustees of its future prosperity.

Cockburn articulated the lawyers' self-conscious image of themselves as an aristocracy of learning as well as of wealth and land:

> The legal profession in Scotland had every recommendation to a person resolved, or compelled, to remain in this country. It had not the large fields open to the practitioner in England, nor the practicable seat in the House of Commons, nor the lofty political and judicial eminences, nor the great fortunes. But it was not a less honourable or a less intellectual line. It is the highest profession that the country knows; its emoluments and prizes are not inadequate to the wants and habits of the upper classes; it has always been adorned by men of ability and learning, who are honoured by the greatest public confidence.[30]

The legal profession's intellectual achievements could serve, therefore, in some degree to compensate for the loss of power and independence suffered by the Scottish ruling class after the Union.

Natural science possessed a special appeal for the Scottish landed and political classes because it exemplified in a particularly clear way the connections between theoretical and material improvement. New understanding of chemical processes could be directly applied to manufacturing and so help to ameliorate society. Because it could serve the demands of the ideology of improvement so precisely, chemistry became the paradigmatic natural science of Enlightenment Edinburgh.[31]

One might account for the demand that gave rise to John Thomson's class in 1799 simply in terms of a continuation of this eighteenth-century tradition of polite interest in the natural sciences, especially in those thought to have technological and economic potentialities. Thomson's introduction to Lauderdale might be compared to the entrée William Cullen gained to influential aristocratic circles through his reputation as a chemist.[32]

Although this argument has a certain plausibility it obscures the degree to which the context in which Thomson operated *differed* from that familiar to Cullen. By 1800 political schism had undermined the high level of consensus that characterized the social and intellectual life of Edinburgh during the mid-eighteenth century. This was evinced in the disruption in 1799 of the Speculative Society. The Speculative was a student debating club founded in 1764 which, with the approval of the Senatus Academicus, met on College premises. It was a typical though outstanding example of the sociable character of Scottish Enlightenment culture: Cockburn described it as 'an institution which has trained more young men to public speaking, talent, and liberal thought, than all the other private institutions in Scotland'.[33] Yet in 1799 Cockburn's Whig friends – Brougham, Horner and Jeffrey prominent among them – set out quite deliberately to politicize this institution at the cost of the secession of many of the older members. 'Political differences ran high at that time', Brougham recalled, 'and there was a personal quarrel with the professors, who had accused us of French principles'.[34]

According to Dwyer this episode 'rang the death knell of the Scottish republic of letters'; and there were contemporaries who lamented the fragmentation of the intelligentsia along party lines that these events announced.[35] The accuracy of this diagnosis can be judged by Cockburn's opinion that 'the *brightest* period in the progress of the [Speculative] society was during the political storm that crossed it in 1799'.[36]

The divisive forces that split the Speculative penetrated deep into the fabric of sociability that had sustained the culture of Enlightenment in Edinburgh. 'It is impossible,' James Gibson Craig recalled,

> to give an idea of the hostile feelings which actuated both parties at this time: society was in a great degree broken up. In ordinary dinner parties it was considered not safe to ask persons to meet who were opposed to each other in politics, and the most extraordinary measures were resorted to.[37]

The society of science, including scientific societies, did not escape the effects of this polarization. In order to understand this politicization of science it is necessary to understand the ideological issues in question. In the process, something of the political significance of scientific endeavour should become evident.

The republican tradition

It is usual to describe as Whigs such leading eighteenth-century Edinburgh literati as William Robertson, Adam Ferguson and Hugh Blair. Inasmuch as these Moderate churchmen were unwavering in their support for the Hanoverian establishment this label is apt. The appellation may, however, give a misleading impression of their general social and political philosophy. This was characterized by a profound conservatism and aversion to all forms of political innovation.

Such conservatism was embodied in Ferguson's historical philosophy. He maintained that both the universe and human history were under direct divine control. The course of events could, therefore, be assumed to have an inherent rationality independent of human determination. Men should defer to divine wisdom and meekly accept that whatever was was for the best. Ferguson's theodicy was therefore also a legitimation of existing political and social arrangements. Although he and his fellow moderates sometimes employed the language of classical republicanism in their rhetoric, 'they rejected virtually every politically progressive proposal and movement of their day, including most varieties of parliamentary, burgh, and ecclesiastical reform, colonial independence, and repeal of the test act'.[38] They were also opposed to the aspirations of the American colonists.

These Whigs had no trouble in accommodating themselves to the Dundas despotism of the last decades of the eighteenth century. And their writings proved serviceable to Tory polemicists in the controversies that followed the French Revolution. They were, in short, outstanding examples of what Pocock calls 'regime Whigs'[39] – eager to serve whichever faction controlled the levers of power and the channels of patronage.

There was, however, an older tradition of Whiggery which had its roots in the political philosophy of the Commonwealth era. These 'Old' or 'Real' Whigs maintained a steady critique of the settlement of 1688 and later of the Hanoverian regime throughout the first half of the eighteenth century.[40] After the accession of George III these complaints against the establishment began to grow in volume and vehemence. They reached a crescendo during the American Revolution and resumed with fresh vigour after 1789.[41]

The programme of the Real Whigs can be reduced to a small number of related principles. Perhaps the most fundamental of these was a rejection of absolute monarchy. While Real Whigs were not necessarily opposed to a hereditary monarch, they did insist that the king be viewed merely as the chief magistrate of the state whose authority derived ultimately from the people, not from divine right. They also maintained that a balance must exist between the various elements of the constitution; if any one organ of the state became predominant, freedom would be endangered. A recurrent Whig lament in the eighteenth century was that this balance was threatened by the growing power of the executive and, above all, by the enormous patronage now available to ministers of the crown. To counter this menace Whigs called for some form of parliamentary reform which would strengthen the popular part of the constitution. Lastly, Real Whigs laid great stress upon freedom of thought. This was especially obvious in their discussions of religious liberties: they were vocal in campaigns to remove civil disabilities on Nonconformists, Jews and Catholics. But more generally, as the eighteenth century progressed the demand for intellectual freedom became secularized, anticipating later liberal formulations of the individual's right to free thought and expression.[42]

Scotland could boast representatives of the Commonwealth tradition throughout the eighteenth century. Indeed, republicanism achieved an institutional foothold in the universities: Glasgow and Aberdeen, in particular, had a reputation for instilling radical principles into their students.[43] When in the 1780s a movement for burgh and parliamentary reform arose in Scotland it drew on Old Whig rhetoric to supply its polemical resources.[44] Archibald Fletcher, for example, saw in the Royal Burghs of Scotland in 1787,

> systems of government, which, by some abuse of language, have obtained the name of *Constitutions*: For they give to the people . . . no voice in the administration; permit persons, once in office, to perpetuate their domination over citizens; afford no adequate redress against the enormities of this power[.][45]

This quotation illustrates how when Whigs sought terms in which to expose the immorality of the existing political order they resorted to the language of civic humanism.[46] The introduction of civic humanism into British political thought in the aftermath of the civil war has been exhaustively described by J.G.A. Pocock.[47] More recently, other scholars have shown the prevalence of this discourse in eighteenth-century Scotland especially in the long-running debates on the cultural consequences of commerce and increasing affluence.[48] Sher, in particular, has shown how the Moderate party in Edinburgh appropriated civic humanist concepts and used them in an essentially conservative way. By the last quarter of the century, however, the same terminology was serving as a peculiarly resonant language of political critique.[49]

Science as virtue

Civic humanism supplied theories both of the state and of personal morality. The two were intimately connected: on the civic humanist view the individual could only achieve liberty and fulfilment through active participation in politics. The moral or just state was the republic because only republican institutions made such political involvement possible. Conversely, the survival of the republic depended upon the integrity of its citizens.[50]

Not every person had the capacity for citizenship. Only the 'virtuous' could aspire to this status; and virtue was dependent, in turn, upon certain contingencies. For Machiavelli the condition of virtue was the exercise of arms; in Harrington and in neo-Harringtonian thought it was the ownership of fixed property.[51] Arms and property were ascribed this enabling status because they ensured the personal *autonomy* of the individual; without this independence citizenship was impossible.

In the course of the eighteenth century this austere conception of virtue underwent considerable modification. Attempts were made to show the compatibility of civic humanist sentiments with the growth of civilization, increased prosperity, and the refinement of manners. Different forms of virtue were appropriate to various stages in the history of society; as John Trenchard expressed it:

> in the first Rise and Beginning of States, a rough and unhewn Virtue, a rude and savage Fierceness, and an unpolished Passion for Liberty, are the Qualities chiefly in Repute: To these succeed military Accomplishments, domestick Arts and Sciences, and such political Knowledge and Acquirements, as are necessary to make States great and formidable Abroad, and to preserve Equality and domestick Happiness and Security at Home; and lastly, when these are attained, follow Politeness, speculative Knowledge, moral and experimental Philosophy, with other Branches of Learning, and the whole Train of the Muses.[52]

This was to invoke an Athenian rather than a Spartan concept of the republic: it supposed a polity in which 'the diversity of [the citizen's] particular attainments heightened his ability to act in the public interest'.[53] In a developed society like eighteenth-century Britain the cultivation of philosophy, both moral and experimental, figured among those civically valuable attainments.

A graphic exposition of this vision of virtuosity as virtue is found in the *Dialogues concerning Education* published in 1745 by David Fordyce (1711–51), the republican Professor of Moral Philosophy at Aberdeen.[54] The hero of the work – Simplicius – travels to an ideal academy to pursue his education. On the journey he remarks upon the richness of the surrounding countryside, noting that 'Such is the influence of liberty, which imploys the naked, and improves the most fertile spots! The happy constitution of Britain may be traced in our blooming fields, as well as in the chearful faces of the inhabitants.'[55]

When Simplicius arrives at the academy (motto: PRO PATRIA), he

> was very agreeably surprized with the sight of so many young gentlemen, some of them of rank and fortune, who were come hither from all quarters to imbibe the principles of science and virtue, in order to qualify for the service of their friends and country'.[56]

Philander, the assistant master of the academy, is presented as a paragon: he is a man of affairs, but

> has read the antients with great taste, and is acquainted with the best modern books: but is particularly conversant with writers on morals and government, to which he adds an extensive knowledge of history; he is an excellent accomptant, and a master of experimental philosophy.[57]

The academy is well equipped with facilities for the latter activity:

> we have a particular apartment for experimental lectures, and a neat apparatus of instruments for all the branches of natural philosophy; it is there Philander gives a very ingenious set of lectures in the experimental way. We have a tolerable laboratory too for chymical experiments, where one Constant . . . performs, and is no mean operator. We have likewise a chamber for dissections, where Euphranor [Master of the Academy] himself frequently performs, and shews us some of the principal parts and functions of the animal system, though he does not pretend to go through a complete course of anatomy.[58]

Chemical Constant is an especially interesting figure. Later we learn that

> Constant is a violent Republican in his principles, and a sworn foe to all tyranny, whether in church or state. So thoroughly has he imbibed the notions of Harrington and Sidney, that you would take him for another Cato. . . . Liberty is his motto, and idol. Hence he goes frequently under the name of the Patriot. For he uses great freedom sometimes with the people in power, and declaims loudly against the growth of corruption, and a general servility, both in principles and manners.[59]

Constant with his ardour for science and love of liberty represents a triumph for the aims of the academy. These were embodied in the initiation new students must undergo. The ceremony takes place in a special chamber at one end of which is a raised throne:

> On the right side of the throne is placed a statue of Virtue; on the left that of Liberty. Above them is this inscription, set in letters of gold, PUBLIC VIRTUE AND LIBERTY. Next the statue of virtue stand a few bustos of some of the most famous law givers of antiquity. . . . On the side of liberty are placed its most eminent asserters. . . . Next the law givers you see a few of the inventors and improvers of useful arts and sciences, among the antients and moderns. On the side of the friends to liberty, are set the heads of some of the most celebrated masters of politics, antient and modern. Among them Plato, Aristotle, Sir Thomas More, Harrington, Sidney.[60]

As if this symbolism was not sufficient to make the point, Euphranor advises candidates

> of the original design of erecting the academy, namely, to instruct and form the youth for being good citizens, countrymen, and members of society; that all its orders and institutions were contrived expressly with this view; – that all their studies and exercises, nay, the whole circle of arts and sciences, are only valuable and honourable, as they are subservient to this grand purpose; – that, henceforth, he is to account himself as part of the public, and made for the good of others; – that he is to consider the train of education, upon which he is now to enter, as a course of instruction and discipline necessary to qualify him for serving the public; – and, finally, that he is a commoner of nature and consequently subjected to the laws and orders of the supreme administration; and is a freeman both in body and mind, and therefore under no controul, but that of reason, and authority founded upon it.[61]

A complex interaction was therefore posited between science and citizenship. On the one hand, the pursuit of science increased an individual's capacity for public service. On the other hand, an ardour for science was one way in which a highly developed civism could be displayed. A similar dialectic was thought to obtain at the societal level; in the history of polities there was an intimacy between the rise of science and the growth of freedom.

It was something of an eighteenth-century cliché that the arts and sciences could prosper only in free societies. Trenchard, for instance, declared that 'The prodigious progress of the *Romans* in Learning, had no other Cause than the Freedom and Equality of their Government.'[62] David Hume subjected this claim to his usual sceptical scrutiny. Hume was prepared to concede that in ancient times it was 'impossible for the arts and sciences to arise, at first, among any people, unless that people enjoy the blessing of a free government'.[63] This was the opinion of the ancient authors such as Longinius who had held that 'the arts and sciences could never flourish but in a free government'. But when *modern* British writers maintained a similar position Hume detected evidence of *parti pris*; authors like Addison and Shaftesbury 'either confined their view merely to ancient facts, or entertained too great partiality in favour of that form of government established among us'. In fact, an impartial observer would recognize that even in modern times absolutist regimes could be hospitable to learning; most notably France, 'which scarcely ever enjoyed any established liberty, . . . yet has carried the arts and sciences as near perfection as any other nation'.[64]

Less sceptical Whigs than Hume saw matters in a different light. James Mackintosh deplored the cultural and intellectual consequences of absolutism. For him the reign of Louis XIV appeared as

> the consummation of whatever is afflicting and degrading in the history of the human race. Talent seemed, in that reign robbed of the conscious elevation, of the erect and manly part, which is its noblest associate and its surest indication.[65]

Mackintosh saw no objection to applying the ancient dictum that science prospered only in republics to recent British history. The Glorious Revolution, he declared, 'deserves more the attention of a philosopher from its indirect influence on the progress of human opinion, than from its immediate effects on the Government of England'. The Revolution

> sanctified . . . the general principles of freedom. It gave the first example in civilized modern Europe of a Government which reconciled a semblance of *political*, and a large portion of *civil* liberty with stability and peace. But above all, Europe owes to it the inestimable blessing of an asylum for freedom of thought. Hence England became the preceptress of the world in philosophy and freedom. Hence arose the generation of sages, who unshackled and emancipated the human mind; from among whom issued the Lockes, the Rousseaus, the Turgots, and the Franklins, the immortal band of preceptors and benefactors of mankind. They silently operated a grand *moral* Revolution, which was in due time to meliorate the social order. They had tyrants to dethrone more formidable than Kings, and from whom Kings held their power. They wrested the sceptre from superstition, and dragged prejudice in triumph. They destroyed the arsenal whence despotism had borrowed her thunders and her chains. These grand enterprizes of philosophic heroism must have preceded the reforms of Civil Government. . . . From this progress of opinion arose the American revolution, and from this, most unquestionably the delivery of France.[66]

John Millar's view of the relationship between intellectual progress and the different forms of government was less polemical and more thoughtful. In his *Historical View of the English Government* (1812) he identified two circumstances that had been favourable to fostering the 'popular part of our constitution'. The growth of arts and manufacturers

> diffused a feeling of independence and a high spirit of liberty, through the great body of the people; while the advancement of science and literature dissipated the narrow political prejudices which had prevailed, and introduced such principles as were more favourable to the equal rights of mankind.[67]

Millar divided the sciences into two main branches: the moral and the natural. The progress of the former had an obvious relevance to politics. As for the latter

> it must be admitted that natural philosophy and the several sciences connected with it, have no immediate effect in extending or improving our ideas with relation to government; further than as all the different branches of knowledge co-operate in dispelling prejudices, in strengthening the intellectual powers, and in promoting an ardent zeal in the discovery of truth.

Natural science could, moreover, exercise an indirect influence on society by improving the processes of manufacture and thus 'promoting opulence and independence in the great body of a people, [which] must contribute, in proportion, to inspire them with sentiments of liberty'.[68]

On the question of the relative scientific performance of France and Britain, Millar took a much more nuanced view than had Mackintosh. It was true that at the beginning of the eighteenth century Britain had outshone France in natural philosophy. But while Mackintosh had ascribed this to the cultural effects of the Glorious Revolution, Millar stressed the importance of individuals: 'Newton . . . produced in this island a rapid advancement of true philosophy; while the high reputation of Des Cartes, in France, gave an unlucky bias to his countrymen, and disposed them to adopt erroneous and chimerical doctrines.' In the course of time, however, this balance was reversed; although

> natural philosophy was thus retarded, it came at length to be more cultivated in France, and in some other parts of Europe, than in Britain; because, from the despotical government in those countries, the inhabitants were, in some measure, debarred from the more generally interesting enquiries upon religion, morality, and politics, and were confined in their speculations, either to matters of taste,

> and abstracted speculation, or to those depending on the nature and operations of corporeal objects.[69]

In the long run, however, it was impossible for such a compartmentalization of philosophic endeavour to endure. In England since 1688

> Philosophy has been constantly advancing in all the departments of science; has been employed in reducing all the works of art, all the appearances of nature, to their principles; and has not neglected to push her researches into political, as well as other branches of speculation.

In consequence of this spread of the scientific spirit, 'The blind respect and reverence paid to ancient institutions has given place to a desire of examining their uses, or criticising their defects, and of appreciating their true merits'.[70] The continental monarchies could not remain forever immune to the spread of enlightenment. While despotism had long kept political speculation in check, 'Philosophy . . . triumphed at length over ancient customs; and the light of science, which had long been diffused in every other department, discovered the rights of man, and the true principles of government'.[71]

I have reviewed the republican tradition and its favoured civic humanist idiom at such length because this complex of ideas and practices provided a normative matrix within which the Whig literati of late eighteenth-century Edinburgh operated. Their politics were much closer to those of the Commonwealthmen than to those of regime Whigs. Their vision of themselves and of their society was, moreover, structured by the discourse of civic humanism: a discourse which, as we have seen, enjoined the pursuit of science on those who sought virtue and within which the extension of the scientific spirit and the growth of liberty were viewed as aspects of the same process of enlightenment.

'Nunquam de Republica desperandum est'

Richard Sher has remarked upon how poorly the literati of mid-eighteenth-century Edinburgh conform to the stereotype of the *philosophe.* They were not impoverished hacks, scribbling away to make a mean living, who inveighed against a hostile social order while dodging the attentions of the civil and ecclesiastical police. The Scottish literati were, with few exceptions, prosperous professional men; they were more accustomed to state patronage than to persecution. 'Their outlook was,' he concludes, 'if not a function of, certainly appropriate to their place as leading members of the liberal professions in a "provincial" society.'[72] We have already seen how conservative and subservient to authority that outlook was.

Conversely, the outlook of the young Edinburgh Whigs of the 1790s can also be seen as 'appropriate' to their place in society – although there might be some argument over whether their social predicament was the cause or the effect of their views. They were also members of the professional elite of the city; but for a period of nearly forty years they lived under a regime that systematically excluded them from patronage and office, and which subjected them to various forms of harassment.

The predicament of the legal Whigs was particularly serious: their very prominence in Edinburgh society ensured that the authorities maintained a specially rigorous control over lawyers. Even as senior a figure as Henry Erskine was in 1796 deposed as Dean of the Faculty of Advocates for daring to challenge government policy. This dismissal, Cockburn recalled, 'was perfectly natural at a time when all intemperance was natural'.[73] The senior Whig members of the Bar were at least secure in their practice; the careers of their younger sympathizers were, however, blighted:

> all hope of official preferment, and even of any professional countenance that power could shew them, was sternly and ostentatiously closed against them. A sacrifice of principle would have relaxed the interdiction; but in no one instance was the sacrifice made or imagined.[74]

The Whig lawyers were regularly reminded of the fate of their fellow advocate Thomas Muir who was sentenced to transportation for his involvement in the movement for parliamentary reform.

The persecution of the Whig lawyers was only a special example of the general repression of Scottish society in the aftermath of the French Revolution. It was not mere rhetoric when John Leyden in 1798 referred to 'the *Terrorists* of Church & State'.[75] The fact that the Whig juniors began their careers 'under proscription, with all its privations and bitterness'[76] goes far to explain the terms in which they viewed and confronted their society.

In his discussion of the varieties of Whiggism Pocock notes that while an 'ideology of modernization' served the interests of the oligarchy, 'the groups excluded from power by the oligarchic regime . . . found it appropriate to adopt an ideology of ancient values, those of the classical republic and its virtues'.[77] The Edinburgh Whigs occupied a position somewhere between these extremes. They were too much the children of the Scottish Enlightenment not to be attached to the ideology of progress – to what Duncan Forbes calls 'scientific Whiggism'.[78] In the hands of Millar and Dugald Stewart scientific Whiggism assumed a much more overtly political character than found in Adam Smith; it became an idiom for the critique of existing social and political arrangements and for the proposal of innovations. While the younger Whigs were often sceptical of Stewart's metaphysics, they attached the greatest importance to his role as a publicist for political economy.[79] But their situation as a persecuted sect under a hateful regime also led them to have recourse to the older – indeed archaic – discourse of classical republicanism.[80]

An attachment to 'the ancient Whig politics of England'[81] is, for example, apparent in Francis Horner's analysis of contemporary politics. He repeatedly spoke of an opposition between the interests of court and country and deprecated the growth of the power of the executive to the detriment of the rights of the people. William Pitt the Younger was cast in the stereotyped role of the domineering 'Minister' responsible for these encroachments on the constitution. Pitt's talents had been 'mischievously employed in devotion to an illiberal unenlightened Court, and after depressing all independence of mind at home, have ruined the power & reputation of the state in its continental relations'.[82]

Horner was, however, no democrat; he showed a deep distrust and contempt for the populace which was no less characteristic of Old Whigs.[83] These two prejudices were combined in Horner's assessment of the likely results of Pitt's repressive policy written in 1795:

> Here it [probably the Treasonable Practices Bill] is very unpopular; even a few of Mr Pitt's advocates, who enjoy a sleep not so profound and unbroken as the others, deem it an unnecessary stretch of power; the violent on the other side reprobate it in that canting phraseology which Rousseau I think invented and the French Revolution made common; while the staunch friends of the Constitution keep it as the happiest measure that could have been devised to hasten the fall of a minister who has brought many calamities on his country, and seems to have formed the design of overthrowing its liberties.[84]

In a subsequent letter to his father Horner revealed his fear that this train of events would lead to the imminent establishment of 'a military monarchy' – a phrase resonant with the Old Whig fear of standing armies.[85]

Alongside the 'stern Tyranny of Pitt', Horner identified 'the vulgar patronage of Melville' (Henry Dundas as was) as one of the principal instruments by which the interests of the court had imposed upon those of the people.[86] He did not disguise his exultation when in 1805 Melville was impeached for misuse of public funds.[87] This deep animus which the Edinburgh Whigs entertained against Melville is explained by their perception of him as a subverter of liberty and a foe to virtue.[88]

Cockburn's indictment of the regime Henry Dundas imposed upon Scotland at the end of the eighteenth century was cast in terms of civic humanism. There is some irony in this: Dundas had himself made adroit use of civic humanist rhetoric to rally support among the landed classes during his rise to power.[89] But by the 1790s, Dundas was 'the Pharos of Scotland. Who steered upon him was safe; who disregarded his light was wrecked. It was to his nod that every man owed what he had got, and looked for what he wished.' Because of his control of patronage and domination of almost every important Scottish institution, Dundas's 'monarchy was absolute'.[90]

Dundas's chief crime was, therefore, that he deprived Scots of their independence, without which there could, in civic humanist terms, be no virtue and no liberty. Such subservience corrupted the individual and ultimately society. Toryism turned men away from their civic responsibilities and made them act 'chiefly on grounds of personal advantage'.[91] Tories were hostile to all forms of popular political participation through which civism could be expressed because they might challenge the dominance of faction; 'we had,' Cockburn lamented, 'no free political institutions whatever'.[92] Scotland under Dundas was therefore the antithesis of the *res publica*: a polity in which there were no citizens, only subjects.

The Whigs were elated even by relatively trivial departures from this state of affairs which permitted some exercise of citizenship. The introduction of a new police establishment in Edinburgh was welcomed because

> *it was the first example of popular election in Scotland*. . . . The gradual extension of the police system over our towns trained the people to expect and to exercise the elective privilege; and the effect of this in exciting and organising public spirit was so great, that the rise of the Edinburgh establishment is one of our local eras.

John Thomson was particularly enthused by this development: he called the new system 'a Divine Institution'.[93]

Thomson was directly involved in other attempts to increase the scope for popular participation in civic matters. He was one of the founders of the New Town Dispensary in 1815 – a measure which 'at its commencement, met with a vehemence of opposition, of which, at the present day, it is difficult to form any conception'.[94] Part of the outcry arose from the proposal that the subscribers to the new Dispensary should elect the managers.[95] Three years later Thomson attempted to assert the right of subscribers to challenge the actions of the managers of the Royal Infirmary of Edinburgh.[96] Since these managers were merely a subset of the clique that dominated the city, this was an attack upon one aspect of that oligarchy in the name of the rights of the wider community. The issue of the alleged mismanagement of the Royal Infirmary was consequently taken up by the liberal press in Edinburgh.[97] Thomson was even accused of being the anonymous editor of 'a violent weekly Paper started here called the Scotsman'.[98]

The pervasive system of political repression had its effect upon the intellectual life of the capital. Looking back on those times, it was

> impossible not to to be struck with the apparent absence of enlightened public views and capacities all over the community. I do not

> recollect a single Scottish work of any permanent . . . value, which even the excitement of that age produced. . . . Indeed the suppression of independent talent or ambition was the tendency of the times. Every Tory principle being absorbed in the horror of innovation . . . , no one could, without renouncing all his hopes, commit the treason of dreaming an independent thought.[99]

To enforce this intellectual despotism a pervasive system of surveillance and police was instituted. Sometimes this system of control was taken to absurd lengths. James Gibson Craig recalled a dinner given in Edinburgh to a score of leading liberals – John Allen and John Thomson among them.

> In the tavern there were two rooms, parallel, separated by a thin wooden partition: what passed in the one room could be distinctly heard in the other. Our party met in the one room . . . and when dinner was served went into the other. After dinner, one of the party . . . left the dinner-table, went in to the next room to get his hat, and almost instantly returned, saying, 'Be on your guard in what you say – the sherrif of the county and a celebrated professor of law [probably David Hume] . . . are in the next room, without wine before them, listening to what is going on.'[100]

Written communication was also subject to scrutiny. Brougham wrote to Francis Horner in September 1797 in the midst of the popular disturbances that followed the imposition of the Militia Act exulting that 'more spirit is manifested than one could have expected'. He added, however, that 'it may be dangerous to speak on these subjects in a letter which will run the risk of being opened at the Post Office – a hint which you may use if you have not already thought of it'.[101]

The clubs and societies which had been centres of free discussion and intellectual vitality in the mid-eighteenth century were special foci of government concern. Why this should be so is evinced by the trend of debate within the Speculative Society in the 1790s. In the early part of the decade a number of daring topics were discussed. On 2 March 1790, for example, the Society debated the question: 'Has the late Revolution in France been equally glorious, and will it be attended with consequences equally beneficial, to that country, that the Revolution in 1688 has been to this?' The question was answered in the affirmative by 6 votes to 4.[102] The following month a much larger majority decided that 'the late Revolution in France [will] have a beneficial effect upon the interests of Great Britain'. While on 29 November 1791 the Speculative determined that there ought to be a parliamentary reform.[103]

John Allen and John Thomson both joined the Speculative on 26 November 1791. They were soon proposing less obviously political, but still incendiary questions for consideration. On 13 March 1792 Allen asked 'Has the belief in a future state been of advantage to mankind, or is it likely ever to be so?' The majority of the Society thought not. A fortnight later Thomson raised the issue of whether 'there ought to be any privileged ranks in society'; this was negatived by 8 votes to 5.[104]

A number of radical motions were still carried in 1793. These included a rejection of the grounds on which Britain had gone to war with France, and an affirmation of the proposition that 'the personal inviolability of the chief magistrate in a monarchical government [is] capable of becoming dangerous to the liberties of the people'.[105] By 1794, however, a reaction had begun. In March the question: 'Is the French Revolution likely to be productive of the extension of civil liberty in Europe?' was decided unanimously in the negative. Finally, in December 1794 political matters were entirely banished from discussion.[106]

So matters rested until 1797 when a younger generation possessed of strong principles began to be heard in the Society, joining forces with some of the existing Whig extremists. In 1799 this grouping – Allen, Brougham, Horner and Cockburn prominent among them – sought to end the ban on political discussion precipitating the split in the Speculative that has already been considered. Even before this episode the Society had again become a forum for the debate of issues too dangerous to be aired elsewhere: William Adam in May 1798 asked James Loch 'what was the subject of your democratical essay, in the "Speculative," and how you dared to say, what I suppose was too true, in a place where Dundas reigns so despotically'.[107]

The Whig coup in the Speculative did not escape the attention of the authorities. In April 1799 a joint committee of the Town Council and Senatus Academicus was formed at the instigation of Robert Dundas, the Lord Advocate, to enquire into the recent proceedings of the Society. The officers of the Speculative were forced to defend themselves against the charge that the Society had become 'a Seminary of infidelity and Sedition'.[108] The committee eventually decided that the threat had been exaggerated and mostly exonerated the Speculative Society. But,

> in respect it appears, that some of its Members have occasionally uttered Sentiments, & employed expressions, obnoxious in point of religious & political tendency, and that the Society by their vote of the 19th february last 'Rescinding all preceding Resolutions restrictive of the freedom of debate,' had given a facility of introducing such sentiments and expressions in future, an admonition should be given to them to be cautious on these points, . . . and to guard with the utmost care against every thing which may have the smallest tendency to weaken their attachment to the principles of the Civil & Ecclesiastical Constitution of their Country.[109]

Even purely scientific associations with no explicit political agenda were subject to the control of the ruling faction. The politicization of Edinburgh science had begun in the 1780s when the Royal Society of Edinburgh was founded by the Dundas interest in the city in order to thwart a rival Whig scheme.[110] In a diatribe against Edinburgh's learned institutions written in 1796 Brougham claimed that the process was now complete, much to the detriment of the value of these societies to science:

> The *Royal Societies* are sunk in a sort of *inertia* – or at least are so much ruled by *party* & what is worse, by *political* party, and still worse, by *aristocratical* politics, – that their labours are useless to science – But granting they are in their zenith; what then? Are young men studying scientific subjects benefited by their institutions? Is *equality*, which ought to be the badge of literary politics, in any degree acknowledged? And do not the very professors in our College, with a *very few* exceptions, discourage every attempt at investigation? From repeated, and peremptory experience I can say, *Yes*[.][111]

Edinburgh science was, in short, 'corrupt' in the strict civic humanist sense of the term: it had ceased to serve the commonwealth and had become subordinate to faction. There was an inversion of the reciprocal relationship that would obtain between science and liberty in the republic. Despotism extended into and vitiated the efforts of the associations formed to advance science and educate the citizen. As a result, young men eager for scientific instruction were thwarted to their own and to society's detriment.

The faults of Edinburgh paled, however, beside the turpitude of St Andrews as recounted by John Leyden in a series of letters to Thomas Brown written between 1797–8. Here too the root of the problem lay in the political and religious subservience of the population. The people of St Andrews were primarly concerned with 'eating, drinking and playing at Cards'. The faculty of the University were especially devoted to these mores: the chief pastime of the professors of Greek, Hebrew, Civil and Ecclesiastical History was whist. Serious metaphysical discussions were strictly proscribed and all forms of scientific intellectual endeavour discouraged: 'Societies of Law Literature, Logic Theology, or Physics, these are plants I am afraid too delicate too [*sic*] vegetate in so rank a soil.' The only scientific investigations that interested the professoriate were those directly related to their lifestyle; the 'learned Dr Rotheram',[112] for instance, 'ever since he caught cold in some hydrostatical Experiments, has been more closely than ever attached to Pneumatics and the Chemical products of the venous fermentation'.[113] The students at this 'wretched College' did not, unlike their Edinburgh counterparts, compensate for professorial shortcomings; there was 'not spirit enough for free Society and at any rate the Students are too much under the controul of the Professors. In Dr

Rotheram's Introductory Lecture he cautioned his Class against foolish Theorists particularly Buffon, Boscovich, and Dr Hutton[.]'[114]

In fact, Leyden found only two individuals capable of 'sensible conversation' in the town. Dr Hunter[115] was 'a man of uncommon merit and ability, and perhaps the most philosophical philologist with whom I have had any acquaintance'. The other – 'Mr Baron' (the Professor of Rhetoric) was also sensible and ingenious; but his virtues were vitiated by the fact that he was 'a ministerial bigot in politics which Dr Hunter does not seem to be'.[116]

Baron's politics, if not his intellectual bent, were typical of St Andrews society. The flourishing cardplaying societies were

> persistently loyal, since Kings and Queens are never out of their hands, on which account it is not surprising that they should often meet with knaves. Indeed I am puzzled to think what the inhabitants will do for Kings and Queens should the present system of Republicanizing go on, for *nunquam de Republica desperandum est.*[117]

The corruption of manners in St Andrews was therefore the result of a pervasive political degradation: 'the lower classes are . . . extremely debauched dissipated and profligate the higher classes are selfish ambitious and deceitful. They are almost all of *loyal mettle,* though perhaps a few might need a political tinker'.[118]

Despite the humourous tone, Leyden's account of St Andrew's society reveals real bitterness and a sense of alienation. His reaction was not, however, one of despair – cultural or otherwise; his response to the frivolity about him was to engage in such scientific pursuits as were available. There was 'perhaps . . . no place where I can spend the Summer more usefully than in St Andrews where there is the very best scope for Botany & where there is access to an excellent Library'.[119] Such endeavours were, however, doomed to frustration in a town where Leyden's passion for science was anomalous. 'There is no chemistry taught here', he complained, 'and no books upon it to be got, except from Dr Hunter, and Brown of Gl[asgow]. So that I have been studying nothing but *conchology.*'[120] Science could only be properly pursued in the society of like-minded men.

Whig science

In the winter of 1795 Brougham approached James Reddie with a proposal for the establishment of 'a sort of *Physical Society,* or rather "Academy." . . . Nothing is more wanted or more desirable.'[121] Brougham's reasons for this plan have already been outlined: the projected society was his answer to the corrupt state of official Edinburgh science. There was, he told Horner,

> an absolute necessity of a society of investigation, considering the degraded state of mathematical & mechanical Philosophy, the inefficacy of *debating clubs* to prevent its fall, & chiefly the abominable politics, trifling pursuits & vile aristocracy which sway the R. Societies of London & Edin^{r}.[122]

The outcome of this initiative was the foundation of the Academy of Physics, which met for the first time in January 1797.[123] The objects of the Academy were to be '*Newtonian Philosophy*, comprehending every subject to which *induction & Reasoning* can be applied – 1. Mathematics, pure & mixed – 2. Physics – 3. Mind – 4. History'.[124]

Geoffrey Cantor has identified the Académie des Sciences in Paris as a possible model for the Academy of Physics. Both institutions shared a meritocratic ideology and an ideal of collective research.[125] But in many ways the Academy of Physics approximated to another exemplar: the imaginary republican academy described by Fordyce.

Fordyce regarded the tendency to form clubs and societies a distinguishing facet of the British national character. One of Simplicius' companions in the Academy confides:

> I had not been long acquainted with these young gentlemen, when we conceived the design of forming ourselves into a club, and having a regular times of meeting, for the sake of conversation. Whether our liberty, or climate, be the reason, I cannot tell; but I found the observation true, that we are, of all nations, the most forward to run into clubs, parties and societies.[126]

Among the many clubs present within the academy some approximated to the goals of the Academy of Physics; they 'seek improvement in mathematical knowledge. . . . Some deal in chymical, and other experimental operations, and by variously subduing and torturing matter, discover its several properties, relations and effects.'[127] Every club 'is a picture of the academy in miniature. The same largeness of enquiry, the same doubting humour, and freedom of debate, prevail in the one as in the other.'[128] A similar egalitarian and liberal regime was enjoined upon the members of the Academy of Physics.

The master of Fordyce's Academy maintained that the experimental method could apply to the moral as well as the natural sciences – as did the members of the Academy of Physics. He further believed that persevering with this method would lead the pupil 'infallibly to the true knowledge of nature and himself; upon which not only a just taste, but the right conduct of life depends'.[129]

This is not to suggest that Fordyce's work had some direct influence on the members of the academy – although they may well have been acquainted with the book. It *is* to argue that the republican values and ideals of Fordyce's imaginary design were also immanent in the constitution of the Academy of Physics. Both shared the goal of enhancing the science, and therefore the virtue, of their members. Where the two *differed* was in the contrasting environments inhabited by the real and the imaginary Academy. While Fordyce's young republicans conducted their studies in a free nation, Brougham and his friends saw their academy as a retreat from a corrupt society. Exiled in St Andrews, John Leyden pleaded for news of the proceedings of the Academy of Physics from his Edinburgh friends.

It is this sectarian character that distinguishes Edinburgh science of the late eighteenth century from that of the previous era; it was one unmistakable sign that the Scottish Enlightenment was drawing to a close. The same partisan aspect characterized a number of other scientific enterprises of the period including John Thomson's chemical class, the chemistry society that grew out of it, and the physiology course that John Allen delivered between 1794 and 1802.

It will be recalled that Thomson began his chemistry course in 1799 under the aegis of James Maitland, Eighth Earl of Lauderdale – an aristocrat with intellectual pretensions. Lauderdale saw himself as, in particular, an authority on political economy; in 1798 he dismissed the argument of Malthus's *Essay on Population* with contempt in a letter to Lord Holland:

> The concept that population proceeds in a Geometrical ratio, and the encrease of Subsistence in an Arithmetical ratio is about one of the most absurd Conceits I have ever chanced to meet with; it would be very fatal in practice, in a family nay[?] perfectly ruinous, to Lady Holland who is about to produce a second it would not be very frightful. Twins are not quite alarming, but to my Wife who has had Nine and who according to this theory ought at the next birth to be delivered of 512 it is seriously frightful.[130]

In 1804 Lauderdale produced a work of his own on political economy.[131]

In Edinburgh during the final decade of the eighteenth century a predilection for political economy often went hand in hand with an interest in chemistry.[132] Brougham remarked of two of his friends that they '[talk] nothing but chemistry and political aconomy [*sic*]'.[133] There was an obvious connection between the two inasmuch as a knowledge of chemistry might lead to improvements in methods of manufacture. In one afternoon Francis Horner recorded that he

> met Kennedy and Thomson, and enjoyed a miscellany of chemical conversation. I went with Kennedy to see the manufacture of tobacco-pipes, which is a very neat operation. A knowledge of the arts, as they are practised in different parts of the country, is what I am desirous

to possess on many accounts; but especially the subserviency of such knowledge to the study of political economy.[134]

Lauderdale's desire for chemical instruction in 1799 was, therefore, a natural extension of his fascination for political economy. Chemistry was besides regarded as a legitimate part of the education of an aristocrat: Lord John Russell went to Edinburgh in 1809 with the intention of attending lectures on chemistry as well as those on humanities.[135] Lauderdale retained his interest in chemistry in later years; he asked John Allen in 1807 for information of Humphry Davy's researches.[136]

Lauderdale was, however, no ordinary improving nobleman. He was a student of Millar with whom he retained close contact throughout later life and from whom he imbibed his political principles.[137] By the 1790s he was regarded as the leader of the Whig party in Scotland. Lauderdale visited France in 1789 and made no secret of his sympathy for the revolutionary cause. Indeed, when he came to Paris in 1806 as part of a peace delegation, Bonaparte is said to have exclaimed: 'comment! on m'envoye un ancien Jacobin'.[138] In domestic politics, Lauderdale was prominent in the radical Whig opposition in parliament and, along with Grey, was the founder of the movement for electoral reform known as the Friends of the People.[139] True to his libertarian principles, Lauderdale had in 1793 interceded with Dundas in an unsuccessful effort to remit the sentence of transportation imposed upon Thomas Muir.[140]

Lauderdale's patronage therefore carried a decided political charge. It was no accident that he chose John Thomson as his chemistry teacher: Brougham remarked in March 1800 that while in Edinburgh, Lauderdale 'associates chiefly with opposition men'.[141] As well as Thomson, these included John Allen of whom Lauderdale entertained 'a very high opinion'.[142] He retained contacts with Thomson and Allen in their later careers, and sought – with varying degrees of success – to secure academic preferment for these protégés (see chapters 2 and 3).

The 'gentlemen of the Parliament House' who attended Thomson's course, as well as engaging in other forms of scientific activity, were, moreover, predominantly drawn from a particular segment of the legal profession. The Scottish Bar, Cockburn remarked, was 'divided into Whigs and Tories, with an overwhelming numerical majority in favor of the latter'.[143] What they lacked in numbers the Whig lawyers made up in talent and accomplishment: in particular, they took upon themselves the responsibility of matching and excelling the literary achievements of earlier generations of Scottish lawyers. Tory members of the profession were, in contrast, less conscious that 'literature . . . is the hereditary fashion of the profession'.[144] They

produced several most excellent men and very respectable lawyers, but not one person, except Walter Scott, who rose to distinction in

> literature, and not one who was looked up to by the country as its guide or instructor in public affairs or in any branch of political philosophy. There never was a period during which in these fields the Tory side of the Bar was so barren.[145]

Cockburn saw the intellectual sterility of the Tory lawyer as a result of his position of political dependence: 'All they had to do was "to maintain the cause of good order'," which meant to resist change, to uphold whatever was, and to abuse as democrats all who differed from them; a task not calculated to liberalize the mind.' On the other hand, those lawyers

> who saw themselves excluded from everything that power could keep from them, reaped the natural advantages of this position. It gave them leisure: persecution cherished elevation of character and habits of self-dependence. Being all branded with the same mark, and put under the same ban, they were separated into a sect of their own, within which there was mirth and friendship, study and hope, ambition and visions.[146]

One way in which members of this sect expressed their solidarity, as well as their distinctness from Tory philistines concerned only with professional advancement, was through their shared interest in natural science.

Cockburn's allusion to the 'elevation of character' and 'habits of self-dependence' that impelled individuals towards such intellectual endeavours is a reminder of the civic humanist codes Whigs employed when seeking to rationalize and ennoble their role in late eighteenth-century Scottish society. Cockburn's image of Edinburgh Whiggery is of a band of heroes. Persecution is almost welcomed as an opportunity for the individual to turn adversity into advantage: to develop personal qualities denied the servile placeman. The real Whig placed the highest premium upon personal integrity as the ultimate bastion against, and reproach to, a corrupt society. The quest for science was prominent among the means by which the individual could attain this heroic stature.

On occasion this heroic role was enacted in a self-conscious and overt way. In the summer of 1799 Henry Brougham joined a group of friends and fellow students on an epic vacation expedition. Their projected destination was Iceland. They were, however, diverted; after travelling through the Western Isles and visiting Orkney, Brougham proceeded to Scandinavia before returning to Scotland in spring 1800.

He wrote several letters to friends and relatives during this voyage which display a curious mixture of styles and preoccupations. One motif is the manners and mores of the various peoples encountered. These are not, however, recounted in a spirit of detached observation. Through a comparison and contrast between these individuals and groups Brougham sought to identify personal and social qualities worthy of emulation or deserving reprobation. In the process he revealed much of his own system of values.

He drew, for example, a sharp distinction between martial virtue, on the one hand, and the the corruption of commerce on the other. During a protracted stay in Glasgow before embarking, Brougham passed his time 'constantly with a set of ten or twelve military men, of long standing in the army, famous for knowledge of the world, and besides, in general, men of the best abilities and temper'. He contrasted the company of these men with the 'golden brutality' of Glasgow which 'served to render our private society doubly agreeable'.[147] Francis Horner (whose father was a merchant) shared Brougham's disdain for mercantile Glasgow, that 'detestable sink of vulgarity and ignorance . . . I would almost as soon go to live at Manchester or Kentucky'.[148]

Brougham's endorsement of military virtue is also typically Old Whig. Horner, though not without misgivings, felt obliged to conform 'to the common sentiments of men in attributing a sort of superior lustre to military glory, which dazzles us in spite of ourselves, and induces us to forget . . . that it has been the scourge of the earth'.[149] The Edinburgh Whigs were enthusiastic participants in the volunteer corps raised during the Napoleonic Wars: in Cockburn's words, 'We were all soldiers, one way or other.'[150]

These attitudes were among the clearest debts the young Whigs of the 1790s owed to the civic humanist tradition in British political thought: a celebration of the martial spirit and an insistence upon the continued importance to society of a citizens' militia can be traced back to the writings of Andrew Fletcher of Saltoun at the end of the seventeenth century.[151] The demand for a Scottish militia had been taken up by the Moderate party at mid-century as an aspect of its essentially conservative political programme.[152] James Mackintosh showed, however, that it was possible to adapt the concept of an armed citizenry to a more progressive political stance.[153]

There was no perceived incompatibility between the practice of arms and the pursuit of science; indeed, the two were thought equally necessary to personal virtue.[154] Brougham in a letter to Robert Lundie conjoined discussion of the proceedings of the Academy of Physics to an account of 'the *Artillery* corps, formed of democrats, freethinkers, Foxites, – & one or two others' to which he belonged.[155] In his journey through the Western Isles, Brougham's party carried weapons; and on at least one occasion he drew his sword in anger.[156] Here, as in Edinburgh, however, he easily combined the martial with the scientific role. As well as cowing the natives by a show of force, Brougham made them the objects of investigation. He referred to the inhabitants of St Kilda as 'the *savages*'; but there was nothing noble about them. After describing their style of life, he concluded that

> Nothing in Captain Cook's voyages comes *half* so low. . . . A total want of curiosity, a stupid gaze of wonder, an excessive eagerness for spirits and tobacco, a laziness only to be conquered by the hope of the above-mentioned cordials, and a beastly degree of filth, the natural consequence of this, render the St Kildian character truly savage.[157]

Brougham attributed the degraded physical and moral condition of these people to the primitive economic conditions of the island. His remarks can therefore be seen as a contribution to the Scottish Enlightenment project of a natural history of man.[158] Brougham however imparted an explicitly political dimension to his analysis of the St Kildian economy attributing much of the blame to the 'present iniquitous method of collecting its produce' and noting the despotic rule that the laird's factor exercised over the inhabitants of the island.[159]

This was only one of several scientific problems that preoccupied Brougham during his voyage. Botany, mineralogy, and geology also figure in the correspondence. These enquiries were, moreover, determined by programmes of investigation formulated among members of his circle in Edinburgh: he wrote to John Allen from Stornoway on 14 August 1799 that

> all my time ashore has been interlarded with inquiries to satisfy, as far as oral information will avail, our scientific queries – Should our expts. not contradict the results of these interrogations, the proof may stand – and at any rate the information thus obtained may serve to direct my own observations & trials – I now send you only notes of results.[160]

These results chiefly concerned the migratory habits of herring. There was also some discussion of mineralogy, but Brougham noted that '*St Kilda* tho' a noble scene for the painter & no uninteresting spectacle to the *moralist* or (rather) *mannerist*, is a very sombre scene for the fossilist'.[161] When on Islay Brougham sent Allen some speculations on the formation of local geological features, leaving botanical and zoological observations to other members of the party.[162]

With the exception of his remarks about the social bases of the poverty of St Kilda, Brougham's expedition might appear as a holiday from politics as well as from the study of law. But the voyage possessed a political meaning which was occasionally made explicit. On 10 August, for example, 'for a frolick' Brougham and his companions 'wore red caps & had ça ira, the Marseillaise &c play'd and chanted in full chorus'.[163] While seven days later Brougham noted 'for the joke we sang the Ça ira'. In both cases the resort to the music and imagery of the French Revolution[164] is presented as a jape. These were, however, frolics that no one would have dared to enjoy in Edinburgh; Brougham's voyage was an escape from the rigid restriction of expression that reigned there. For a while he was part of an untrammelled society: 'freedom of speech reigns among us' he declared.[165]

Such liberty could, however, only be temporary. By March 1800 Brougham was back in Edinburgh: he had abandoned his design of visiting St Petersburg because of the 'extremely disagreeable situation of travellers residing in Russia . . . Contrary to my expectations – I found despotism the more hideous the nearer I attempted to approach it.'[166] Brougham turned his attention to John Thomson's plan for a new Chemical Society; he had no doubt that 'common prudence, and a moderate share of ardour, must ensure its victory over all rivals'. He also acknowledged the demands of professional study upon his time: both he and Horner intended to pass their Bar examinations that summer.[167] In such a combination of intellectual endeavours the individual could find freedom even under despotic rule.

A liberal education

In November 1796 Brougham sent Horner an assessment of various possible candidates for membership of the Academy of Physics. In the process, he revealed much about his view of which intellectual characteristics were to be most esteemed. The various strengths and weaknesses of individuals were subjected to rigorous scrutiny. William Gillespie, for example,

> has an accurate knowledge of Chemistry & Natural History – & a very tolerable acquaintance with *Physics* – But his *forte* is that sort of *Physiology*, and mixture of Anatomy with metaphysics, in which *Darwin* shines. Like him too, Gillespie excells in *fancy*: has strong inventive powers [and] is a good poet. But he follows the Philosopher of Derby into his faults; wants steadiness – & is . . . too fanciful in his theories. This account may satisfy you that he will make an excellent member – tho' not just a good *founder*.[168]

Other candidates were faulted for lacking in knowledge of particular departments of science. William Erskine 'has applied more to Metaphysics & Belles lettres than to physical subjects'. This defect could, however, be remedied by a course of reading and attendance on John Robison's lectures. Brougham had no such reservations about the qualities of James Reddie who 'joins the good qualities of *every one* – Languages Politics – Law. Metaphysics & Physics – & History are almost equally his own & in all he is *original* & *true* when he pleases.'[169]

Breadth of learning was therefore clearly a prime good for Brougham. This erudition needed to be complemented by the capacity for original thought; but fancy must in turn be disciplined by an adherence to sound rules of reasoning. Intellectual independence was also highly esteemed: James Lang was praised because

> On *all* subjects to which he attends he thinks for *himself* – & to almost all his knowledge *extends*. He began to *think* about 6 years ago – for till then he lived with a *seceder*. His thoughts took a total change – for till then they were those of a *Calvinist* – his opinions are now free, yet (I hope & think) true; for he has *studied, Berkeley, Rousseau* & *Hume* –[170]

Lang was thus, in every sense of the word, a freethinker.

Brougham's scale of intellectual values owed obvious debts to the real Whig tradition and to the civic humanist ethic. A man's independence was prized in the field of philosophical endeavour as much as in his overtly political opinions and actions. Independence might imply freedom from external or internalized constraints upon thought: in Lang's case this required emancipation from the trammels of religious dogma. Independence might also, however, be construed as *autonomy* – as an individual's ability to think and judge on a wide range of subjects without needing to defer to the superior wisdom of another. This desideratum helps to explain the extent of the studies that Brougham and his colleagues felt obligated to pursue.

Their ambitious and demanding educational programme can be seen as a response to anxieties about the possible effects of the growth of knowledge and increased specialization upon the individual. These fears emerged from the eighteenth-century discussion of the wider implications of the tendency towards an ever greater division of labour in society. According to John Millar, the same process at work in the organization of manual labour also impinged upon more intellectual occupations:

> Even in the cultivation of the sciences, the circumstances of society have commonly occasioned a separation of certain learned professions; and diverted . . . the attention of numerous classes of men to particular departments of knowledge. The diseases and accidents by which health is impaired have given rise to the medical profession, with its respective divisions, connected with various branches of natural science.[171]

Millar had no doubt that 'this division in the labours, both of art and of science, is calculated for promoting their improvement'.[172] Like Adam Smith, however, he apprehended that this socially beneficial process of differentiation might pose dangers for the individuals involved. Although

> the separation of different trades and professions, together with the consequent division of labour and application in the exercise of

> them, has a tendency to improve every art or science, it has frequently an opposite effect upon the personal qualities of those individuals who are engaged in such employments.[173]

What was threatened was the 'general knowledge' of a population who increasingly ran the risk of becoming confined to one area of life, or one field of study, having little acquaintance with what lay beyond. Such restriction could have grave psychological effects; at worst, in the case of manual workers:

> As their employment requires constant attention to an object which can afford no variety of occupation to their minds, they are apt to acquire an habitual vacancy of thought, unenlivened by any prospects, but such as are derived from the future wages of their labour, or from the grateful returns of bodily repose and sleep. They become, like machines, actuated by a regular weight, and performing certain movements with great celerity and exactness, but of small compass, and unfitted for any other use.[174]

Francis Horner in 1800 bore witness to the accuracy of Millar's prophecy. The working men he encountered were 'in general mere machines, and not unfrequently more ignorant, literally speaking, than the tools which they employ'.[175]

In Millar's view those engaged in the sciences and liberal arts were not in the same degree of danger; certain necessary aspects of their occupations mitigated the worst effects of specialization. In all the

> liberal occupations or scientific professions, there are certain principles to be studied by every person engaged in practice; principles which admit of an extensive application to a variety of objects, and which, in many cases, cannot be properly applied without exercising the united powers of imagination and judgment.[176]

Through their possession of these general ratiocinative principles the upper classes were able to cultivate and enjoy the full range of arts and science; and Millar hoped that their cultural influence might serve to ameliorate in some measure the ignorance and stupidity of the manual labourer.[177]

This discourse about the moral consequences of the division of labour can itself be seen as a refinement of a much older civic humanist concern that professional specialization might impair the individual's capacity for virtue. Specialization compromised the autonomy of the citizen; inasmuch as he relied upon another to perform some essential function, a man became *dependent* upon that specialist. There was clearly a dilemma here: the division of labour, the very force that ensured the growth of civilization, was also 'a prime cause of corruption'[178] Ultimately, specialization posed a threat to the integrity of the self.

Millar suggested one way in which this challenge could be confronted and managed. He argued that underlying the diversity of knowledge and attainments in the modern world there remained certain general principles which possessed a universal applicability. Anyone who commanded those principles was enabled to grasp the systematic connections binding together the different departments of art and science. He might even aspire to a measure of theoretical and practical competence in several of those fields.

For Dugald Stewart the primary aim of a 'liberal education' was to impart these capacities to the student: 'To abridge the labour of reasoning, and of memory, by directing the attention to general principles, instead of particular truths, is the professed aim of all philosophy.'[179] Men of 'general views' possessed, he declared, a 'natural superiority . . . over the common drudges in business'.[180]

The foundations of this outlook lay for Stewart and his pupils in a grounding in metaphysics.[181] English observers of Scottish intellectual life were often bewildered and sometimes exasperated by this emphasis. Sydney Smith complained that the Scots were 'more fond of disputing on mind and matter than on anything which can have a reference to the real world'.[182] While Lord John Russell, who had himself attended Stewart's lectures, felt that

> Moral Philosophy tho' a very pretty amusement, seems to me to consist chiefly in confuting the very absurd errors of those who have set themselves up as very cognoscent in the human kind, & I who had never heard of those opinions & consequently never been a convert to them am not a bit wiser than I was before.[183]

Horner in 1800 sought to convince another English aristocrat of the injustice of such scepticism about the practical value of the science of mind: in any attempt to reform scientific language, he argued,

> The foundation of the great fabric must unquestionably be laid in metaphysics; or to abandon so alarming a phrase, in that science which teaches us to analyse the operations of the understanding, and to resolve complex ideas into their simple elements.[184]

In his account of the educational value of metaphysical studies, Stewart emphasized that 'those individuals who are habitually occupied with them cannot fail to acquire a more than ordinary capacity of withdrawing their thoughts from things external, and of directing them to the phenomena of mind'. This imparted both a certain mental dexterity and an ability to subject common assumptions to critical analysis: 'Hence an accuracy and a subtlety in their distinctions on all subjects, and those peculiarities in their views, which are characteristical of unbiassed and original speculation.' But perhaps

> the most valuable fruit they derive from their researches is, that scrupulous precision in the use of language, upon which, more than upon any one circumstance whatever, the logical accuracy of our reasonings, and the justness of our conclusions, essentially depend.[185]

Stewart did not, however, enjoin *only* metaphysical studies upon his students; he saw grave drawbacks attached to an exclusive concern with introspection. His pedagogic goal was to produce good citizens – men of affairs not mere contemplative philosophers. General principles derived from abstraction could only be successfully applied to the business of life by those who also possessed 'a certain degree of practical and experimental skill'. Such skill involved

> a talent for minute and comprehensive and rapid observation; a memory, at once retentive and ready; in order to present to us accurately, and without reflexion, our theoretical knowledge; a presence of mind, not to be disconcerted by unexpected occurrences; and, in some cases, an uncommon degree of perfection in the external senses, and in the mechanical capacities of the body.[186]

These capacities were only to be acquired amid 'the active scenes of life'.[187]

To avoid the inconveniencies attendant upon the mere metaphysician, Stewart therefore exhorted his students to counteract the tendency to excessive abstraction by means of 'other studies'; these would direct the student's attention toward the observation 'not only of physical phenomena, but of the character and manners of the society around him'.[188] The natural sciences (the study of society included) could serve to supply the deficiencies of pure metaphysics. Scientific endeavour provided a theatre in which theory could be applied to the understanding and manipulation of the material world. Only through such praxis could the individual acquire the range of capacities that fully fitted him for life.

While Stewart enjoined students to pursue a wide range of scientific and literary pursuits in order to avoid the dangers of specialization, he also warned in 1827 against the contrary error:

> This caution I conceive to be particularly necessary in the present times, in which there is a manifest bias in the rising generation to consider knowledge rather in the light of an accomplishment, subservient to conversation, than of a solid acquisition, convertible to purposes of real and permanent utility.[189]

What distinguished the acquirements of the truly educated man from the magpie accumulations of the mere dilettante was that the learning of the former was founded upon a knowledge of the general principles that underlay all science.

Such an education equipped a man for citizenship. It helped secure his autonomy against the encroachments of specialization. The system of *Lernfreiheit* obtaining in the University of Edinburgh made practicable attempts to explore science in all its aspects. John Leyden, for instance, 'availed himself of the unlimited freedom bestowed by the regulations of the College in making himself acquainted with every branch of liberal science'.[190] Although formally a student of divinity, Leyden attended a variety of courses during his time as a student in Edinburgh, in the conviction that 'whoever confines his studies to Theology, will neither excell in that science nor in any other'. In his first three years he restricted himself 'in Sciences, to Criticism, Moral & Natural or Mechanical Philosophy'. Subsequently, 'I . . . attended lectures on Natural History, Chemistry & Botany, w[h] with the different branches of Anatomy, Surgery, Medicine & Physiology have chiefly occupied my attention these three last years'.[191] Such attendance on medical classes as part of a general education was not unique to Leyden; in 1798 he asked his fellow divinity student, Thomas Logan, 'Are you studying Mathematics along with Anatomy and attending the Infirmary[?]'[192]

In his lectures, Stewart simply assumed a familiarity with medical theory among his students. He remarked, for example, that 'in the political system, as well as in the animal body . . . there is a sort of *vis medicatrix,* which is sufficient for the cure of partial disorders'.[193] Elsewhere he wrote at length about the epistemological bases of medical practice.[194] In the case of his best-known disciples, Stewart was fully justified in making these assumptions.

Medicine, Cockburn recalled, had 'great attractions' for Francis Jeffrey, 'and for a short time he studied it'. His friendship with John Allen and John Thomson and other medical Whigs also enabled Jeffrey to gain a 'desultory acquaintance with their science. One way or other, he at least learned enough about it to make him generally a fanciful sufferer and a speculative doctor, when he himself was the patient.'[195] Although Cockburn was more amused than impressed by such pretensions to medical erudition, philosophic Whigs were serious in their assumption of medical competence. Most notably, Francis Horner took a keen intellectual interest in the protracted illness that finally killed him. Allen wrote to him detailing the opinions of various physicians on the pathology of the case; and Horner presumed to draw his own conclusions. Shortly before his death he confided to his father: 'I have long considered it a settled point, that my complaints were not consumptive.'[196]

The converse of the refusal to acquiesce in the rigid demarcations of specialism was an insistence that an individual's own professional persona should be founded upon philosophic principles. Horner again supplied the clearest example of this conviction in action. On the eve of his return to Edinburgh in October 1797, Horner had determined upon a career at the Scottish Bar; he had also decided that 'It ought to be the main object of my ambition, and the point of tendency for all the thoughts, exertions, and labours of my life, to become a consummate lawyer, both in practice *and in science.*'[197] He took for granted that law was a science, not merely a practical art. Law therefore had certain principles in common to all sciences; its study could, in consequence, be enhanced by the mutual illustration and reinforcement to be derived from the pursuit of *other* sciences. Indeed, it was only this approach to law that made it a worthy calling for the citizen. When in 1802 Horner transferred to the Bar in London he was scathing about the intellectual and ethical stature of his new colleagues:

> in general, the lawyers of this place are extremely ill-informed; slaves to those habits, which in our profession more than any other, are illiberal and fatal to intellectual activity as well as moral independence. They seldom know any thing out of the second; they can only labour on a brief; and I believe their habits become at last so morbid, that a certain application to the palm is the only stimulus by which their powers of mind can be excited.[198]

Metaphysics was fundamental to the enterprise of the scientific lawyer: 'it is only on a complete and scientific knowledge of human nature and the theory of morals, that the path is laid towards the elements of legislative science'. The science of politics, as embodied in history, was also of obvious relevance.[199] Natural sciences too had their part in Horner's plan from the outset: Horner told John Hewlett soon after his return to Edinburgh that

> beside the civil law lectures . . . I propose to go through a course of chemistry and natural philosophy. . . . I shall from time to time do myself the pleasure of troubling you with letters, and I please myself with the expectation of having my labours in Justinian, Newton, and Lavoisier, agreeably relieved by your communications.[200]

In the spring of 1798 Horner began a journal in which he painstakingly recorded his efforts to come to grips with the 'formidable problem' he had set himself: 'To unite the business of a Scotch lawyer with an ardent and steady pursuit of science, as well as the cultivation of taste, especially in composition.'[201] This journal has something of the character of a secularized Puritan diary. There is the same ardent striving for an unattainable goal coupled with a merciless self-criticism. The deity that Horner tried to satisfy was not, however, the Christian God, but science; the object of desire not grace, but knowledge. At the end of the first year of the journal he lamented that

> but a small proportion of this twelvemonth has been employed in study, and that small portion by no means so well employed as it might have been. Instead of a regular plan, my reading has been extremely desultory; the consequence of which is, that instead of having got a firm footing on any part of the field of *science*, I have only a recollection of its form and appearance, from having once been there; instead of having made any approaches towards a systematic possession of the knowledge that I have, it lies scattered through my memory in a mass of unarranged particulars.[202]

In May 1799 Horner attempted to regularize his studies. He divided his objects into four categories: 'Law, Physical Science, Political Philosophy, and English Composition'. Under the second of these headings, he planned to confine himself to attending 'Allen's lectures on the *Animal Economy*, in order to acquire some general notion of a subject on which I have at present no knowledge whatever.'[203] In order not to interfere with his other commitments, he undertook, however, to do no reading on this subject except before breakfast. On 2 May Horner duly

> Got up two hours before breakfast, and read some of 'Bell's Anatomy', on the Mechanism of the Heart: this opened a scene of wonders to me. I consulted Allen what books I should previously read to get a general knowledge of as much physiology as I shall need in order to follow his lectures.[204]

Horner also took an interest in current developments in geology: after exploring Salisbury Crags with John Playfair, he wondered 'Am I in the fulness of time to become a convert to the Huttonian heresy? – at present, perhaps, *excitabilis superstitio*, as Tacitus calls Christianity.'[205] The religious metaphor for scientific innovation is noteworthy.

The journal makes it clear, however, that Horner's real passion was for chemistry. At times this predilection threatened the strict discipline he sought to impose upon his diverse intellectual labours. Indeed, on occasion he spoke of his chemical pursuits as a form of sensual self-indulgence which should engender feelings of guilt. Thus 20 May 1800 was 'given up to a chemical debauch'; 26 May 'Another day of chemical dissipation'; while on another occasion Horner confessed: 'I was more idle today, as to Scots law, than I have been for a fortnight past: an experiment in chemistry led me astray, *sinner that I am!*'[206]

The special interest of philosophic Whigs in chemistry has already been noted: it was manifested both in their attendance on Thomson's course and in the subsequent formation of the Chemical Society.[207] This may seem to need no explanation. Chemistry was a very popular pastime among the educated classes in Edinburgh as elsewhere at the turn of the nineteenth century; in 1800 Thomas Charles Hope, the Professor of Chemistry in the university, was obliged to ask the Town Council for funds to erect a new gallery in his lecture theatre because 'the number of students who attend the Chemical class, has been greatly increasing and is in this year in particular so great, that there are not seats enough to accommodate them'.[208] Philosophic Whigs were, however, contemptuous of this fashionable pursuit of chemistry and of other sciences; Jeffrey noted that 'in the informed circles of society, a man can scarcely pass current without knowing something of political economy, chemistry, mineralogy, geology, and etymology'.[209] After attending some of Davy's lectures at the Royal Institution, Horner remarked that 'The audience is assembled by the influence of fashion merely; and fashion and chemistry form a very incongruous union.' He conceded, however, that such gatherings did represent a 'trophy to the sciences'; he approved especially of 'the association of female and masculine minds in the pursuit of useful knowledge'.[210] But *his* engagement with chemistry, and that of his peers, was altogether more profound than that of Davy's audience or of such to whom Hope's lectures might appeal.[211]

There were special reasons why chemistry at the end of the eighteenth century might appeal to Whigs. The dramatic transformation the science had recently undergone testified to the dynamic nature of knowledge and to the potential for intellectual innovation. Even John Millar, who usually showed only a desultory interest in the physical sciences, 'for a whole winter, thought of nothing but chemistry' after Lavoisier produced 'his astonishing experiments, and no less astonishing system built on these experiments'. Millar's biographer makes clear that it was the systematic aspect of Lavoisier's achievement that provoked this admiration and fascination.[212] The fact that the chemical revolution was primarily a French achievement itself gave this knowledge a powerful political charge.

For Horner the particular appeal of chemistry lay in the scope it gave for the fullest accomplishment of Stewart's educational programme. Through chemical studies one could apply and enrich those general principles that were essential to a philosophic approach to all aspects of life. Chemistry was, therefore, a paradigmatic science to be studied as a source of intellectual edification in the individual and as a means of facilitating progress in other departments of knowledge.[213] These assumptions were evident in the advice Horner gave his brother in 1803:

> With respect to chemistry in general, I would advise you, from my own experience, not to throw away many hours upon manual and operative experiments; because your plan of life will not admit of your ever

> becoming a perfect, or even a tolerable, workman. Indeed your views should be a good deal higher than that. . . . Do not imagine that I am disposed to damp your ardour for chemical studies; on the contrary, my design is to promote it, by urging you to choose the most important and most difficult part of the science. Do not quit it, till you have mastered all the general knowledge, that has hitherto been ascertained, of the chemical phenomena of nature: and have fixed in your mind such a store of facts, and principles, and *reasonings*, as will enable you, after you turn your labours to other subjects, to follow the future discoveries and improvements that may be made. Only remember, that an evening, for your purposes, may be far more profitably employed in labouring to comprehend a general theory or exposition of great natural phenomena, or to detect the fallacy of an inaccurate hypothesis, than in watching the manipulation of a process which you perfectly understand, but which you cannot qualify yourself perfectly to execute. You have to render yourself a man of liberal information and of a cultivated understanding, not a dexterous apothecary.[214]

What was 'sinful' about Horner's own chemical activities was that he sometimes forgot these injunctions and pursued the subject in a frivolous way with more regard to the sensuous pleasures its operations could bring than to the loftier goals of intellectual edification. He wrote of an experiment he witnessed as 'beautiful'; and on another occasion confessed that 'chemical manufactures [are] my principal amusements'.[215] He later repented these indulgences:

> I often reflect, with pain and regret, that the hours I have wasted in distilling sulphuric acid for future experiments that never were attempted, might have put me in the full and steady possession of the doctrine of latent heat, the theory of affinities, that of oxygenation in its various branches, &c., &c.[216]

Among the general principles that might be elucidated by the study of modern chemistry, Horner laid special stress on the implications of the chemical revolution for philosophical language. In the course of a correspondence with the Duke of Somerset, he acknowledged the desirability of a 'real character' – a special scientific code free from the defects of ordinary language. 'It is not so much as an abbreviated record of our knowledge already ascertained,' he wrote, 'that the improvement of philosophic language is so desirable, as because it would facilitate farther discovery and farther generalisation.' This was as true of political economy and metaphysics as of natural philosophy. The one science in which a reform of linguistic manners had already occurred provided a promising precedent:

> What was done by the French chemists affords a most flattering example; yet I suspect it was conducted with a considerable portion of empirical good luck, rather than upon comprehensive views of philosophic logic. It is to this great speculation that I look for the improvement of Science.[217]

Horner's celebration of the possibility of creating a new scientific language upon a priori principles was also an endorsement of the possibilities of a rationalistic approach to problems of all descriptions. He thus subscribed to what Edmund Burke saw as one of the worst aspects of the revolutionary ethos: the belief that it was possible – indeed, desirable – to discard the experience of the past as embodied in institutions and usage and to begin anew. In contrast, John Robison was much more cautious in his assessment of the new French chemical terminology; Lavoisier, he claimed, had through pride acquiesced 'in measures which may be called violent and unbecoming. As for the *imitatores, servum pecus,* they boggled at no incongruity with common language and sentiment; and rather had a pride in it as mark of their authority over the opinions of other men'. Robison's own notion of how science might be improved was distinctly Burkean in tone:

> The same principles, and the very same men, formed this nomenclature and the new kalendar and metrical system of the French. But these inconveniences are not essential to a good systematic nomenclature. Had all the proper names been retained, and had a becoming deference been paid to ordinary language and sentiment, the nomenclature would have been much more intelligible, would be free from paradox, – and Mr Lavoisier's well deserved honours would have been fully secured to him.[218]

Robison's suspicion of the new chemical nomenclature was much more typical of British reactions than was Horner's enthusiasm.[219]

Somerset responded to Horner's recommendations by asking how he might acquire some grounding in chemistry 'for the purpose of examining the principles upon which the modern nomenclature of that Science has been contrived'. Horner advised that for the general scholar 'a very adequate idea may be acquired of the chemical theory and terminology, without submitting to the inconvenience of performing a single experiment personally'; it was, however, necessary 'to *see* some other person exhibit a considerable number of experiments'. He therefore recommended the Duke to seek the assistance of some of the London chemists. With the aid of such instruction Somerset would be able to examine 'with reference to the introduction of similar improvements into other branches of philosophy, the principles upon which the chemists have invented their own language'. The efforts of the French chemists were defective inasmuch as they were '*unprincipled*'; a rigorous logical analysis was required to distinguish the judicious part of their invention from error.[220]

Horner's correspondence with Somerset on these topics was voluminous. The pains he took are some indication of the importance he attached to fostering the scientific interests of a politically active member of the aristocracy. There was more at issue here than merely some hope of personal advancement; the Whig tradition emphasized the importance of the involvement of this class of person in philosophy. Among the advantageous circumstances that the students enjoyed in Fordyce's imaginary academy was that

> gentlemen of the first rank, in the town and neighbourhood, do us often the honour to visit our academy, and think it not beneath them to take a part in our free familiar conversations, and to give us their assistance and advice, particularly in making experiments. To their favour our master recommends us with a peculiar warmth and tenderness.[221]

Beside whatever patronage and protection such individuals might offer, it was important for Whigs to inculcate correct philosophic principles into the minds of sympathetic aristocrats in order to promote reform. Intellectual and political innovation were seen as closely conjoined. Horner took the opportunity of his letters to Somerset on the improvement of scientific language to make this point explicitly:

> can we indeed flatter ourselves with much hope of success in these splendid projects of philosophical innovation, when we observe the fate of some plans of improvement which have every appearance of practicable sympathy, and of which the necessity is undeniably most imperious?

He alluded to a bill to reform the law on enclosures that Somerset had recently failed to steer through parliament. There was, Horner declared, no rational basis for the opposition to this measure: 'The repositories of old prejudice must be ransacked for such objections.'[222] He declared himself

> mortified, tho' very little surprised, to find the dignatories of the Law, ranging themselves with those of the Church, in opposition to salutary innovations. But it is indeed too hard a task to yield up inveterate habits, and at the end of a life exhausted in obedient reverence of Established rules, to attempt the speculative examination of their reasonableness and justice.[223]

Hence the importance of instilling rational principles at an early age into those destined to direct the affairs of the nation. An exposure of this class to the science of political economy in the course of their education was perhaps the most obvious means of securing this end. But *all* science, inasmuch as it exemplified general philosophic axioms, could be considered a branch of civics. In 1803 Horner wrote to his brother that:

> When I was at Oxford last week, I attended an evening lecture on *Galvanism* . . . by Dr Kidd, the reader in chemistry . . . It was exactly what it was intended to be, popular & interesting; adapted to the capacity of young gentlemen commoners, among whom I was pleased to see germinating lords & embryo statesmen attending with apparent satisfaction & diligence.[224]

For Horner, science retained its old Whig status as a school for citizenship.

Conclusion

To understand philosophic Whiggism it is necessary to locate the utterances of the individuals who constituted the phenomenon within a grid of values and meanings formed by several intersecting lines of discourse. These cultural flows structured the philosophic Whig's view of himself as a social actor; they formed the basis of a normative system which supplied him with goals and aversions; they provided him with a rhetorical language with which to justify himself and his allies and to characterize the depravity of his enemies.

A number of key polarities dominated the verbal universe of the philosophic Whig. He organized his vision of society about such contrasts as: citizenship/subjection; autonomy/dependence; liberty/servitude; reason/prejudice; science/ignorance. All these were, however, modalities of the fundamental antithesis between virtue and corruption.

Because an ardour for science possessed for much of the eighteenth century an acknowledged status in real Whig ideology as one means by which a man could affirm and reinforce his virtue, its pursuit became a political act. Amid the intensified anatagonisms of late eighteenth-century Edinburgh the significance of such acts became more profound. The need to affirm one's virtue was all the more urgent in a polity where 'A country gentleman with any public principle except devotion to Henry Dundas, was viewed as a wonder, or rather as a monster.'[225] To the Whig intellectuals forced to live under this regime, scientific endeavour was one strategy against corruption. Those like Allen and Thomson who possessed specialized scientific knowledge were valued within the Whig community because they could facilitate these efforts; in sharing their knowledge they were also imparting virtue to their fellow citizens.

The fervent pursuit of science might also be seen as a displacement of energy that, under different circumstances, would have been directed into professional or more overtly political activities. But the quest for knowledge and self-development was not an alternative to these other aims. Horner's case, in particular, shows how science could be conducive to the creation both of a professional persona and propaedeutic to statesmanship.

While biding their time, the Whigs were not wasting it; they shared Dugald Stewart's vision of education as a preparation for the task of political renewal they would one day be called upon to undertake. They took to heart his ringing exhortations:

> Surely, if any thing can have a tendency to call forth in the public service the exertions of individuals, it must be an idea of the magnitude of that work in which they are conspiring, and a belief of the permanence of those benefits, which they confer on mankind by every attempt to inform and enlighten them. As in antient Rome, therefore, it was regarded as the mark of a good citizen never to despair of the fortunes of the republic; – so the good citizen of the world, whatever may be the political aspect of his own times, will never despair of the fortunes of the human race; but will act upon the conviction, that prejudice, slavery, and corruption, must gradually give way to truth, liberty, and virtue[.][226]

Given such assumptions, the pursuit of knowledge was itself a political act, a step on the road to reformation: 'if truth and virtue be diffused', Thomas Brown maintained, 'their own silent operation may gradually succeed in producing that very amendment, which mere force . . . would have failed to effect'.[227]

Appendix 1

Chart showing the participation of prominent Edinburgh Whigs in scientific activities

John Allen (1771–1843)	M	CS		
Henry Brougham (1778–1868)	L	AP	CS	
Thomas Brown (1778–1820)	L/M	AP	PC	
Francis Horner (1778–1817)	L	AP	CS	PC
Francis Jeffrey (1773–1850)	L	AP	CS	
John Leyden (1771–1811)	D/M	AP	PC	
John Archibald Murray (1779–1859)	L	AP		
James Reddie (1773–1852)	L	AP		
John Thomson (1765–1846)	M		CS	PC

Notes: L = Law; M = Medicine; D = Divinity; AP = Member of the Academy of Physics; CS = Member of Chemical Society; PC = Member of John Allen's Physiology Class.

2

John Allen, physiologist and Friend of the People

Introduction

John Allen is usually supposed to have lived two quite discrete lives. After qualifying as a surgeon in Edinburgh and acquiring a considerable reputation as a teacher in the extramural school of medical education, he abandoned the profession of medicine in his early thirties for more literary pursuits. In 1802 Allen joined the household of Lord and Lady Holland, first as their physician, later as librarian and general factotum. In this latter incarnation Allen has a secure, if minor, place in the writings on Holland House, that early nineteenth-century centre of Whig politics, desultory cultural exchange, and endless dinner parties. Leslie Mitchell maintains that Allen did much to give Holland House 'a reputation for unrestrained, even farouche, ways of thought'.[1] One of the Holland children left a memorable verbal portait of Allen at this period of his life: 'He was a stout, strong man, with a very large head, a broad face, enormous round silver spectacles before a pair of peculiarly bright and intelligent eyes, and with the thickest legs I ever remember.'[2]

Assessing Allen's post-1802 career Henry Cockburn acknowledged that his alliance with the Hollands showed him

> most of Europe well; and introduced him, confidentially, to the best society in England. The transition from this to the private political line was natural; and in this line there is no one man whose talent and learning is of so much use to his party.

But Cockburn added that 'all this latent importance, dignified luxury, and indirect usefulness was obtained . . . at far too high a price when it lost him the glory of being the first medical teacher in Europe'.[3]

Cockburn was clear on why Allen did not achieve the professional status that would have enabled him to play this role: 'Had not his political opinions made it prudent for him to despair of being ever allowed to adorn our

College, he would probably have remained here . . . and had a great reputation.'[4] Allen's foreshortened career as a physiologist was therefore a product of his other persona during his years in Edinburgh: that of an advocate of controversial and, in the eyes of some, subversive political causes.

The Friend of the People

According to Cockburn, Edinburgh society at the end of the eighteenth century was dominated by a single preoccupation:

> Everything rung, and was connected, with the Revolution in France; which, for above 20 years, was or was made, the all in all. Everything, not this or that thing, but literally everything, was soaked in this one event.[5]

The Revolution in France gave fresh impetus to the movement for reform which had arisen in Britain in the second half of the eighteenth century. This association between domestic reform and foreign revolution was to have grave consequences. All those who promoted even moderate plans of political innovation were indiscriminately branded 'Jacobins' by an increasingly frightened establishment; for those labelled in this way, the implications were serious.

The Society of the Friends of the People was founded in April 1792 by a group of Foxite Whigs led in parliament by Charles Grey. The Society sought to steer a middle course between outright rejection of reform on the one hand and, on the other, an increasingly vocal radical movement represented by the Society for Constitutional Information and the London Corresponding Society. The main plank of the platform of the Friends of the People was a call for some measure of parliamentary reform; they argued that only if the establishment yielded something to the demands of the disenfranchised could a British revolution be avoided.[6]

Its name notwithstanding, the Society was by no means a democratic body. 'The people' were only those thought by virtue of their education and ownership of property to be entitled to a place in the political nation. A discrepancy had arisen between existing forms of representation and the legitimate aspirations of members of this class. When this defect had been remedied, however, the great bulk of the population would remain without a vote.

A number of provincial societies calling themselves 'Friends of the People' were formed throughout the country in the latter part of 1792; the Edinburgh Society was pre-eminent among them. These societies tended to be more radical than Grey's prototype; Paineite doctrines had spread quickly throughout the country, and especially in Scotland.[7] The Edinburgh Society contained, however, a wide variety of opinion: it included extreme democrats as well as advocates of cautious electoral reform.

The authorities kept an anxious eye on the activities of the Friends of the People from the outset. The Lord Advocate advised Dundas that around 200 had attended an inaugural meeting on 28 August 1792 at the Barber's Hall. He noted that 'they correspond with the Jacobins in France, and with the London Corresponding Society'. Worse still were the sentiments expressed by members of the Society at a subsequent meeting: one member 'spoke as follows – "It is a maxim of mine that a King should be sacrificed to the Nation every 100 years."'[8] Later reports presented a less alarming view of the goals of the Society; its chief ends were said to be 'A compleat and general Reform of the Burrows . . . [and] a Reform of the Excise Laws.'[9] By the beginning of November Dundas was advised that 'no less than thousands' had joined the Society, but reassured that 'many of these detest the idea of a revolution'.[10]

There was, however, sufficient evidence to convince the government that the Friends of the People was a potentially revolutionary force. An anonymous member of the Glasgow Society sent Dundas – along with a copy of their resolutions – a note that ended: 'Fame, Sound the downfall of *Monarchy* and the elevation of . . . *Democracy*.'[11] The Friends of the People were thought dangerous for two principal reasons. They consorted with a foreign and potentially hostile power: the Edinburgh Society was reported in September 1792 to be considering a petition to parliament calling on Britain to declare war on France's continental enemies.[12] Moreover, the Societies represented a dangerous alliance between dissident members of the political nation and the lower orders. A Glasgow notable expressed these fears in a letter that found its way to Dundas. 'The Success of the French Democrats', it was alleged,

> has had a most mischievous Effect here – did it go no further than give Occasion for Triumph to those who entertain the same Sentiments here, there would be little harm for they are very few in number – and but two of them possessed of any considerable Influence and Respectability – but it has led them to think of forming Societies for Reformation into which the lower Class of People are invited to enter – and however insignificant these Leaders may be in themselves, when backed with the Mob they become formidable.[13]

Intercepted letters from William Reddie, a grocer who belonged to the Edinburgh Society, appeared to provide a link between the external and internal threat. After outlining the aims of the Friends of the People, he concluded that 'it must end in a Republic – The Soldiers will not fight against the people but should they France will send 80,000 to help us . . . we will not hesitate which to choose a Civil war or Slavery.'[14]

John Allen was involved in the liberal politics of Edinburgh at least as early as the summer of 1791 when he helped organize a dinner at the

Fortune Tavern to celebrate the French Revolution.[15] According to one of his close associates from this period, Allen was an 'enthusiastic admirer of Mr Fox, and of the *first* proceedings of the French revolution, which appeared to us to promise the greatest blessings to mankind'.[16] Allen's friend and fellow medical student John Thomson was also present at this gathering. By the end of 1792 Thomson had, however, distanced himself from the more extreme forms of political agitation then emerging in Edinburgh. He unsuccessfully advised Allen to do the same: in November 1792 a mutual acquaintance wrote to Thomson that 'Allen has left the hospital, but notwithstanding your good advice, is still by far too deeply engaged in democratic politics'.[17] By this date Allen had joined the Friends of the People, and seems to have been engaged in an attempt to moderate the influence of the '*volcanic* heads' – notably, the advocate Thomas Muir – who had assumed the leadership of the Society.[18]

Whatever misgivings Allen may have had about the direction of the Society, he attended the First General Convention of the Delegates of the Societies of the Friends of the People held in Edinburgh in December 1792. Government spies took notes of the proceedings of this gathering and informed their masters of the alarming language adopted by some of the delegates, who, for instance, addressed one another as 'citizens' in clear imitation of French precedents. Despite such rhetorical flourishes it is clear that the delegates were not revolutionaries; indeed, they were at pains to affirm their loyalty to the British constitution and to distance *their* calls for reform from the demands of those who were ready to use force to secure political change.

Allen's recorded contributions to the proceedings conform to this pattern. The government spy noted that on 12 December 'Mr Allen made a motion, which he read in so low a voice that we could not hear it.' The official record of the Convention gives this motion as:

> That in order to supersede the necessity of constantly resorting to the aid of a military force, it be recommended by the Convention to the Associated Friends of the People, in the different parts of the country, to hold themselves in readiness to support the civil magistrate when required for the suppression of any popular tumults that may arise in their neighbourhood.[19]

The following day Allen elaborated upon this proposal. He moved 'that we should hold ourselves in readiness to assist the Civil Magistrates in suppressing all riots and tumults and the Associations should be properly provided with Arms for that purpose'.[20] This time the spy did hear what Allen said. Another delegate took up the suggestion with enthusiasm: he proposed that 'every associator should be provided with what is commonly called a *Brown Janet*, with Powder Ball and Bayonet to be ready to assist in quelling every appearance of riot and Sedition'. Others opposed the motion, however, and after some discussion, Allen withdrew it.[21]

These interventions can be viewed (as Allen probably intended that they should) simply as attempts to demonstrate the loyalty of the Friends of the People and their opposition to any form of violent revolution. They may also be seen as evidence of Allen's subscription to the familiar civic humanist doctrine that an armed citizenry was the best guarantor of the constitution. But this call to arms would confirm the authorities in their worst suspicions about the seditious intent of the Society. When Sherrif Pringle forwarded the minutes of the meeting to Dundas he remarked upon the 'very extraordinary motion made by a Mr Allan'. Despite his involvement in the Fortune Tavern gathering, this seems to have been the first occasion that Allen became the object of the authorities' serious attention – Pringle was uncertain whether he was a Writer to the Signet or a medical student. Ominously, however, he undertook to 'get full information' on Allen and other delegates involved in the discussion.[22]

Allen's name does not figure in the list of delegates to the Second General Convention of the Friends of the People held in April and May of 1793. This was probably because of his disaffection with the tendency of the Society in this later period. Delegates to the second Convention tended to be of lower social standing than before. Although divisions persisted, the radicals gradually gained the ascendancy; in particular, they fostered links with the more extremist London Corresponding Society. In November a further Convention passed motions in favour of universal suffrage and annual parliaments – measures which Allen would have abhorred.[23]

Allen therefore seems to have dissociated himself from the Friends of the People before the authorities finally suppressed the movement for parliamentary reform. By the end of 1793 the Scottish Societies had moved far beyond any programme of reform compatible with his Whig principles.[24] From the point of view of Allen's professional prospects, however, the damage was done. W. Russell in his letter to Thomson had apprehended that Allen's political activism would have this result: 'I have constantly urged him to *give out,* as I conceive it is not only inconsistent with his present situation, but occupies his time, and introduces him to a public notice which, at best, can be of no advantage to him'.[25]

Junior Whig lawyers found it difficult to establish themselves at the Bar during these years in the face of official disapprobation. Allen seems to have faced similar difficulties when he tried to set up in practice. His resort to teaching in the extramural school was, in part, an attempt to secure an alternative source of income and to establish a public reputation. It was not, however, impossible for a medical Whig to succeed in Edinburgh. John Thomson was said by 1817 to enjoy 'a practice among the Jacobins here equal to £2000'.[26] The source of this statement was hostile to Thomson; the size of his income and the character of his patients are therefore open to some doubt. What *is* clear, however, from this and other sources is that Thomson, despite his politics, succeeded in practice while Allen failed.

This difference may be explained in part by the fact that Thomson wisely stayed aloof from the Friends of the People; he was in London at the time of the first Convention and on his return to Edinburgh was careful to avoid even casual association with notorious reformers.[27] Second, Thomson was a far more adroit professional politician than Allen. He cultivated powerful members of the Royal College of Surgeons, such as Benjamin Bell. He took their side, and that of James Gregory, in the dispute at the turn of the century over the organization of the surgical service at the Royal Infirmary.[28] His reward was to be one of the six surgeons-in-ordinary appointed to the Infirmary in 1800.[29]

Allen had also favoured reform of the system of surgical attendance. The issue could be understood in terms of Whig principles: Cockburn presented the Gregory–Bell controversy as a struggle between public welfare and the private interests of a particular sect.[30] Although on this occasion these principles prevailed (albeit by accident), Allen lacked either the acumen or the inclination to reap any personal benefit from being on the winning side.

He was also bereft of the social graces requisite for professional success. In 1795 Allen, writing under the pseudonym 'Necessitarian' published a critique of James Gregory's views on causation.[31] Thomson, according to Gregory, 'knew and approved of the composition and publication' of this pamphlet, in which 'I was reproached, in very bitter and sarcastic terms, with gross ignorance, bad reasoning, and shameful disingenuity'.[32] While Thomson, however, managed to maintain civil relations with Gregory, 'From that time to this [Allen] has not once spoken to me, or appeared even to know me when we meet in the streets, as we have done very often; and I dare say he never will speak to me again'. Gregory's claim that he, none the less, bore Allen no ill will and 'should be very glad to have an opportunity to convince him of that by doing him any good office in my power'[33] is difficult to credit.

By 1803, when Gregory wrote these words, Allen had left Edinburgh. But he left behind memories that militated against any return. Early in 1804 the chair of natural history in Edinburgh University became vacant. This was a regius chair which had in the past been the object of competition between political factions in the city.[34] When the new vacancy occurred, the Whig party in Edinburgh abetted by their allies in London set about securing the election of a professor sympathetic to their cause; their chosen candidate was John Allen – then in Spain with Lord and Lady Holland.

The Earl of Lauderdale and Dugald Stewart attempted to muster support for Allen at Edinburgh,[35] while in London Francis Horner took the lead. On 5 January 1804 Horner wrote to James Loch – an old Speculative

Society associate of Allen – urging him to 'Think of all the possible channels of Scotch patronage and application; & come to town soon tomorrow that we may concert together.' He was quite open about the political motives behind the canvass. The vacancy had occurred when the hold of the Dundas faction upon Scottish patronage had loosened; the attempt to appoint a Whig professor of natural history was to be considered 'another try against Lord Melville'. The rival contender was no less the creature of faction: 'for [Robert] Jameson, under the old govt. was assured of the reversion'.[36]

Because the object of these manoeuvres was a regius chair, the final decision lay with the ministry in London. In 1804 Henry Addington was Prime Minister – a fact that gave Allen's supporters some hope. Although Addington was no friend of the Whigs, he was hostile to Melville and opposed to his dominance of Scotland; he might therefore be reluctant to appoint the previous administration's chosen candidate.[37] Allen's supporters may have been encouraged by the appointment in 1803 by Addington's administration of the Whig James Russell to be Regius Professor of Clinical Surgery. By 7 January Horner felt able to tell Thomson that 'we entertain a very sanguine hope of Allen's success, we were all in high spirits yesterday about it. With [Sydney] Smith, Brougham, &c we drank full bumpers to the event.'[38]

These celebrations proved premature. Horner had solicited the aid of Sir James Mackintosh on Allen's behalf. He was an especially important ally because, while 'he never has had, & would not have any political connection with the present people,' Mackintosh did have the opportunity of an interview with Addington at which he agreed to press Allen's claims. He found that Addington was already aware of Allen's candidature for the chair of natural history; in the course of the ensuing discussion, the reasons for his ultimate failure emerged. Avoiding all reference to party politics, Mackintosh presented the matter

> as a public measure of a literary nature, in which he was warmly interested; both by what he knew of Allen's high merits, and by his attachment to the University in which he had been educated – That that University had suffered much of late years by an absurd System of hereditary professorships, and by several unfit nominations of the Town Council – that the present was an occasion on which Govt. might introduce one of the ablest & most scientific men in the kingdom, and that it would be honourable to the King's Govt. to shew that in their department at least the appointments were influenced by that consideration.[39]

Addington listened to this appeal with 'much attention and observed that Tierney[40] had already spoken of Mr Allen to him in the strongest terms of approbation'. It became clear, however, that 'He must have heard of him . . . from *other* quarters; for he asked Mackintosh, whether Allen was sound in matters of religion & politics; and whether he had not in the late times shewn some violence in these respects'. Mackintosh did his best to deflect these accusations; and Horner remained optimistic of success. He recognized, however, that 'it is of much importance to us that the matter sh^{d} be decided as soon as possible. If the cry of atheism & Jacobinism becomes very loud against us, it will frighten the doctor [i.e. Addington].'[41]

It became evident that this cry against Allen was loudest from the quarter of Edinburgh. Brougham found support there for Allen from such as James Russell, Professor of Clinical Surgery, and Andrew Dalzel, the Professor of Greek. But when Brougham made advances to John Robison, Professor of Natural Philosophy, he found that 'with the greatest opinion of [Allen's] talents . . . – I fear he thinks him illuminated.'[42] Robison had in 1797 published his *Proofs of a Conspiracy against all the Religions and Governments of Europe, Carried on in the Secret Meetings of Free Masons, Illuminati, and Reading Societies.* In this work he argued that atheist *illuminati*, working through masonic lodges, had fomented revolution in Europe.[43] By hinting that he thought Allen 'illuminated', Robison was placing him among this dangerous group of subversive intellectuals.

Jameson was, in contrast, considered safe by both the Senatus Academicus and the Patrons of the University. When on 4 January 1804 the Town Council considered the question of the natural history chair, they received 'the strongest recommendations in his favour from the Principal and a number of the Professors of the College'. The Council accordingly resolved unanimously to recommend Jameson for the appointment.[44]

Lauderdale and Stewart's canvass for Allen was countered by a campaign for Jameson orchestrated by Charles Hope, the Lord Advocate, in conjunction with George Baird, Principal of the University. Both were staunch Dundas men. Hope wrote to the Home Secretary on 6 January that 'I am very earnestly solicited by my Constituents, the Lord Provost, Magistrates & Council of the City of Edinburgh, to recommend Mr Robert Jameson' for the natural history chair. He felt the need to defend these constitutents from any charge of nepotism in the matter; they were

> motivated by no motive but the public good – I know that Mr Jameson is not connected with nor related to, a single Member of the Council, & that they have espoused his Interest merely from the testimonials they have received from the leading Members of the University of his abilities as a Naturalist.[45]

These included Thomas Charles Hope (chemistry), James Home (materia medica), and – despite his Whig credentials – John Playfair (mathematics).[46] By way of further recommendation, the Lord Provost despatched a resolution in favour of Jameson from the Highland and Agricultural Society of Scotland.[47]

Nowhere in this correspondence is there any direct reference to Allen. When, however, Baird came to add his own voice to the chorus in favour of Jameson, he made what may have been an indirect allusion to the rival candidate. Apart from his other qualifications, Baird declared that Jameson

> entertains those sound & rational principles in both morals & Religion which will lead him to employ those favourable opportunities which a Professor of Natural History possesses of supporting by his doctrines the interests of piety & public Virtue – a consideration, which will strike most impressively, those who have seen most clearly the modes which have been adopted & are adopting for the corruption of manners & of opinion upon the Continent.[48]

Even Allen's most fervent supporter could not suggest that *he* was a proponent of 'sound' religious principles; it was, on the contrary, all too easy to insinuate that he was of the party that had corrupted European manners and opinion.

The crown bowed to this pressure from Edinburgh. On 20 January Charles Yorke, the Home Secretary, ordered his staff to 'render an appointment to be made out for Mr Robert Jameson, who is recommended by the Ld. Advocate'.[49] Joseph Banks (who had supported Jameson) had remarked to Yorke early in the contest, 'I know that a man in your Situation is too often forced to sacrifice the best Candidate to the superior interest of a less promising one.'[50] On 14 March 1804 Jameson's commission as the new Professor of Natural History arrived.[51] Allen's aspirations to the chair were passed over in silence.

Allen's abortive attempt to return to Edinburgh makes a number of points. It shows the strength of the hostility to him in Edinburgh. This antipathy rested on a perception of him as a particularly dangerous kind of political animal: one of a species of radical intellectual who threatened the stability of the social order. On the other hand, Allen's supporters advanced his cause not only because he was of their party, but also because of genuine admiration for his achievements in medical science. In order to understand both these perceptions, it is necessary to study Allen's scientific utterances as a student and teacher in Edinburgh.

Remarkably, Allen never published any extended statement of his views on natural science. His scientific opinions need to be reconstructed from manuscript sources. Two of these are of particular importance: the dissertation on mania Allen delivered to the Royal Medical Society in 1790; and the lectures on the animal economy that he gave as an extramural teacher between 1794 and 1802.

The physiology of the human mind

The Royal Medical Society was the descendant of a student association formed in 1734. It had received a royal charter in 1778 through the efforts of Andrew Duncan senior. The members of the Society presented dissertations for their own improvement and for the edification of their colleagues. New ideas were evaluated and old doctrines were criticized within the Society, which also supplied facilities for experimental investigations. The Royal Medical Society therefore provided medical students with a valuable alternative to the limited and dogmatic instruction offered within the university.[52]

The Royal Medical Society was noted for its egalitarian procedures and organization. By the end of the eighteenth century its debates had, moreover, assumed a quasi-political aspect. 'We mimicked,' James Mackintosh recalled, 'or rather felt all the passions of an administration and opposition; and we debated the cure of a dysentry with as much factious violence as if our subject had been the rights of a people, or the fate of an empire.'[53] This tendency of student medical societies to becomes cockpits was deprecated by some senior members of the profession. James Gregory maintained that

> It is much to be lamented, for the sake of the science, and the art of Physic in all its branches, . . . that this unlucky analogy of politics has of late been so much attended to, while the more just and strict analogies of other sciences and other arts have been totally overlooked.[54]

Gregory also decried the dismissive attitudes to scientific authority that membership of such societies inculcated.[55] The contrast between Gregory's attitude and that of his predecessor William Cullen is illuminating. Cullen, in true Enlightenment fashion, had encouraged questions from and discussion with his students, Gregory reverted to a more authoritarian model of pedagogy in which communicative flows were to be far more strictly controlled; there was no proper role for the student except as auditor.

Moreover, the technical medical issues in question themselves became politicized, especially in the course of the Brunonian debates of the 1770s and 1780s. Michael Barfoot has remarked on how the Brunonian conception of the body in health corresponded to republican notions of a sound polity.[56] Even under the despotic regime of the 1790s, the Royal Medical Society retained a considerable degree of independence and daring: in March 1792 its members adopted a provocative motion on the issue of slavery:

> All men are born free and equal in rights. The first object of government is to secure to *all* the right which *all* derive from nature to *civil*

liberty. The object of *political* liberty is to prevent the abuse of power in government[.][57]

Allen's contributions to its proceedings reveal that the Royal Medical Society also continued to provide a platform for 'dangerous' views that challenged some of the most cherished beliefs of orthodoxy.[58] The dissertation on mania – probably given late in 1790[59] – was purportedly a clinical treatise. Allen maintained, however, that

> I have always thought it impossible for any one to compose a proper dissertation on the Pathology of a disease, without prefixing to it his ideas on that branch of Physiology, which is related to his subject; or at least, without specifying the particular system he adopts.[60]

Before one could arrive at a pathology of the human mind, a requisite was 'a general view of the functions exercised by the Organs immediately concerned in the production of Mind'.[61]

By framing the question in these terms, Allen made a number of crucial assumptions: notably, that there *were* organs the function of which was the production of mind. The implication was that the study of mind and its diseases should be seen as part of physiology – the science of the living body, of what Allen called 'the moving solid'. All the phenomena of animal life were, he maintained, reducible to sensation and contraction; for a mental physiology the former was the key vital property.

All sensations, Allen declared, 'are the immediate consequence of certain changes taking place in the Brain'.[62] He went on to suggest how mental phenomena might be represented in the substance of the brain. Specific brain fibres were assigned to the reception of particular sensations and fixed connections existed between them.

> From these connexions established between the fibres appropriated to the different Sensations, we are to explain the phenomena of Memory & Imagination. In the former, the ideas follow the exact order which the original Sensations kept; in the latter the utmost latitude is allowed. But even in the wildest reveries of Imagination, there is still a connexion preserved between the different ideas, which succeed each other.[63]

Allen referred to an observation of Hume that in various languages certain simple ideas tended to be connected together, 'so that the complex terms of one language correspond with and can be translated into those of another'. Allen saw this as 'A certain proof that the simple ideas, expressed by these complex terms, are bound together, by some universal principle, which has an equal influence on all Mankind.'[64] This universal principle could lie only in the organization of the brain.

Allen also saw a physical basis for Hume's constant-conjunction theory of causation. He acknowledged the validity of the claim that 'it is only from one object constantly following another, and being in exact proportion to it, that we call the first, *Cause*; the second, *Effect*'. Allen then turned to 'the nature, and cause of the Belief' in a regular conjunction between cause and effect. It was evident that repeated experience of a conjunction between two experiences would create a firm connection between the fibres in the brain that received these sensations:

> Hence . . . the presence of the one object occasions a more clear, steady, and vivid conception of the other, attended by more considerable emotions. This appears as distinct an explanation, as can possibly be given, of the mode of conceiving objects, which we call Belief.[65]

Allen went on to challenge the notion that volition was the efficient cause of voluntary motion. Within his scheme of physiological psychology this could only be so if the will could effect changes in the matter of the brain: without such change no bodily movement could occur. But,

> no sentient, and intelligent Being can act, without being conscious of acting . . . Now I ask any Man, whether he is conscious of producing that change in his Brain, which Reason, and experiment inform him, must precede Voluntary Motion. I know he must answer in the negative. He produces, then, according to the Theory hitherto received, a certain effect, without being conscious of producing that effect; nay, without being able, by the strictest attention, to perceive its existence. His mind, therefore, the sentient and intelligent Principle said to reside within him, is no more to be regarded as the Author of that effect, than of an action committed at the distance of three Thousand Leagues.[66]

The 'obvious, though, I confess, extraordinary conclusion presents itself. *That voluntary motion is never to be regarded as the effect of volition*'. Since, however, the will was the only mental faculty that had ever been ascribed a role in the causation of motion, 'The latter must, therefore, depend on some corporeal Cause.' The efficient cause of voluntary motion, as of sensation, memory, and the association of ideas, must lie in the 'Mechanism of the Brain'.[67]

In order to explain how this mechanism might work, Allen proposed what was in effect a reflex theory of the action of the nervous system. 'Let us', he wrote,

> conceive an Automaton, or Figure, which shall perform all the actions of a Man, and possess his internal organization, and outward

> appearance, without being endowed with Sensation. The impressions of external objects on the organs of this Automaton shall produce there certain changes which by means of a connexion with the moving fibres, through the medium of the Brain, shall be followed by certain actions. And the effect of these actions shall be, in general, the preservation of the Automaton from danger, and the procuring of such impressions as shall tend to prolong its existence, or multiply its species. The Automaton shall be of such a nature as to undergo a permanent change from the impression of objects, so that the effect of new impressions shall be modified by preceding ones. Connexions between different fibres shall be formed, so that a renewal of motion in one shall be followed by a renewal of motion in others; and these connexions shall be regulated by fixed laws. . . . Let this Automaton be endowed with Sensation, and it shall become a Man.[68]

Within this scheme voluntary action was explained mechanistically. At first the automaton would have no volitions; but,

> after it has been affected with different Sensations, some will prove more agreeable to it than others; these it will prefer; and from the mechanism already established, it shall happen, that the actions, which please it most, or which have the greatest tendency to procure it happiness, shall in general, be performed.

Because of this association between certain movements and desired sensations, the automaton 'shall think itself the Author of these Actions, and assume the attributes of *Liberty*'. For Allen, 'Man is exactly this Automaton, possessed of the faculty of Sensation.' The effects ascribed to human intelligence could, therefore, be understood in purely naturalistic terms: they were to be 'classed along with the labours of the Bee, the growth of a Mushroom; or the Crystallization of a Salt. Fixed and invariable they are governed by the laws of Mechanism.'[69]

Under the pretext of a discussion of mania, Allen thus reduced the human mind to a physical phenomenon. He did not draw out the implications of his theory for ideas of the immateriality and immortality of the soul. He did, however, comment upon the consequences of his doctrine for natural theology:

> Here let me reflect a moment on the conduct of those Pseudo-Philosophers who contemplating the similitude between the works of art, and the productions of Nature, have presumptuously insisted, that, because, in their opinion human Intelligence is the cause of Art that, a similar Intelligence must, of necessity, be the productive Cause of Nature. Such a mode of reasoning must be given up if the present theory be adopted.

> Since it would be absurd to attempt explaining the production of Nature, by analogical reasoning from Art, the cause of the latter being equally unknown; and erroneous to ascribe it to a principle, which, in the latter case has been proved not to exist.[70]

After which, the discussion of the pathology and therapeutics of mania with which Allen concluded his dissertation comes as something of an anticlimax.

The dissertation on mania was primarily an attempt to demystify the human mind. Allen undermined the idea of the mind as an immaterial being which somehow manipulated the body. In its place he put a mechanistic concept of sensation and motion in which consciousness played no causal role. In so doing, Allen challenged prevailing notions of liberty; and any such move was seen as a threat to prevailing ideas of the conditions of morality. Dugald Stewart wrote in 1793 that all his enquiries 'concerning the moral constitution of man, proceed on the supposition, that he has a freedom of choice between good and evil'. Stewart recognized the existence of a contrary philosophy entertained by

> a few speculative men, who have contended, that the actions we perform are the necessary result of the constituents of our minds operated on by external circumstances; and what we commonly call moral delinquencies are as much a part of our destiny, as the corporeal or intellectual qualities we have received from nature.[71]

Speculations on this subject could, Stewart continued, 'hardly fail to affect very materially both our conduct and our happiness'.[72] From his strictures upon Hartley, Darwin and Priestley it is evident that Stewart considered invalid *any* attempt to jumble together 'scholastic metaphysics and hypothetical physiology'.[73]

Allen held, moreover, that the supposed analogy between the human and divine intelligence must be abandoned, and with it the argument from design. Not only did he therefore place himself alongside the sceptical Hume and psychological materialists like Hartley, he also allied himself with such infidels of the Enlightenment as La Mettrie and Holbach.[74] There are grounds for believing that Allen's reputation for atheism was justified.[75] He was not alone in adopting such extreme views; many of his student contemporaries were of like mind. Moreover, such philosophic radicalism had strong political implications. Dugald Stewart explained that there was good reason for the emphasis he had placed upon the doctrines of natural religion in his Edinburgh lectures after 1792:

> The danger with which I conceived the youth of this country to be threatened by that inundation of sceptical or rather atheistical

publications which were then imported from the Continent, was immensely increased by the enthusiasm which, at the dawn of the French Revolution, was naturally excited in young and generous minds. A supposed connection between an enlightened zeal for Political Liberty and the reckless boldness of the uncompromising freethinker, operated powerfully with the vain and the ignorant in favour of the publications alluded to.[76]

Stewart's own endeavour was to show that a zeal for liberty could be combined with a philosophically and religiously safe stance. Soon after his arrival in Edinburgh however, Allen was, without equivocation an 'uncompromising freethinker'.

The animal oeconomy

The lectures Allen gave in the Edinburgh extramural school between 1794 and 1802 are the basis of his place in the canonical history of Scottish medicine. They are usually presented as the first course given in Edinburgh devoted solely to physiology. Allen himself described his course as on the 'Animal Oeconomy' – a Hunterian expression. The course should not, however, be viewed solely in terms of the history of medical education; it was a cultural event of much wider significance. Allen kept careful class lists which reveal the kind of students he attracted. In all, 53 students attended the course, several taking it more than once. These included students of medicine and a number of senior members of the profession; but there was also a substantial contingent of non-professional auditors. The rump of the Whig party in Edinburgh was well represented.[77]

In an undated notebook, presumably composed while preparing his first course of lectures, Allen sketched his ideas on the scope and nature of physiology. He sought initially to distinguish physiology from other cognate departments of science:

> The Anatomist, Chemist, natural Philosopher & Metaphysician consider ye animal System as related to their respective subjects – the Physiologist considers these subjects as related to the living System as they enable him to describe & explain the condition of the body and mind, which are necessary to life, and health – the *mind* to have a place, only so far as distinctly referable to ye state of ye body.[78]

Physiology was thus distinguished from metaphysics. In his lectures Allen respected this distinction. He did in 1795–6 give an extended critique of Thomas Reid's theory of vision;[79] this could, however, be legitimately regarded as a topic where mental phenomena were 'distinctly referable to the state of the body'. Later teachers of physiology in Edinburgh were less careful of this boundary: John Thomson's lectures on the institutes of medicine in the 1820s contained extensive discussion of metaphysics (see chapter 4).

Allen showed little interest in the relations between physiology, pathology and clinical medicine. In view of the fact that physiology was traditionally taught in the Edinburgh school in conjunction with pathology and therapeutics as the component parts of the 'Institutes of Medicine,'[80] this was a significant innovation. Occasionally, Allen did suggest that the phenomena of disease might cast light upon normal function and vice versa. Thus the elaboration of heat in the body during fever was 'a direct Proof of the *Caloric* there produced being derived, from the Combustion of the absorbed Fat'.[81] Conversely,

> An analogy between the funct^{ns} of the skin and those of the lungs might be founded on the phenomena of their diseases, as Catarrh & Pneumonia; from the oper^{n} of diff^{t} remedies; and on the similar^{y} in each of the aqueous exhal^{n}[.][82]

Very rarely Allen referred to his own clinical experience to make some general point; he recalled, for example, an anomalous case where the patient, 'a young woman of a corpulent habit, [who] passed through a fever attended with very little augment^{n} of heat; & it was observed that after the disease, her body had suffered no sensible emaciation'.[83] In general, however, physiological discourse was for Allen distinct from the language and concerns of the practice of medicine.

Allen also demarcated physiology from anatomy. This was, in part, because of a conviction in the limited value of the study of structure to the resolution of physiological questions: 'All the assistance afforded by the *present state* of Anatomy to the Theories of Secretion consists in ascertaining the diff^{t} Vesicles with w^{h} the blood passes thro. organs destined for the diff^{t} Secretions.'[84] Allen also seemed to defer to some tacit division of labour within the Edinburgh medical school. When speaking of absorption, for instance, he remarked that 'This function is so much the object of discussion in the Anatom^{l} Theatre that it shall be here treated very briefly.'[85] The mechanical part of respiration was similarly 'so much the peculiar Province of Anatomy & is so generally known that it shall not here occupy much Attention'.[86]

At a more profound level, however, the physiologist's concerns were distinct from those of the anatomist because physiology dealt only with the *living* body. Indeed, its province was the phenomenon of life itself – to which structural considerations were at most secondary. There was in Allen's scheme no single centre that could be identified as the seat and source of life: it had been proposed by some

> to take [the animal oeconomy] in ye series of Cause & effect, but this is not practicable without a deal of hypothesis – Is ye Brain ye main spring of ye Machine & yet its operations cannot subsist an instant without muscular Contraction – Is it then ye muscular fibre? It is doubtful whether a single contraction w^{d} be obtained without ye nervous matter dispersed through ye substance of ye muscles. Is it the nervous extremities then? their condition is modified by that of ye vessels of ye brain – So that we return to ye point from which we set out –[87]

Life, therefore, was equally diffused through the constituent parts of the body; these cooperated to form an interdependent and indivisible whole.

Elsewhere in these preparatory notes Allen appears to diverge from this principle by giving a heuristic, if not a causal, priority to the nervous system. All the functions, he declared,

> involve moving powers – muscles depend on nerves – nerves on ye brain – ye Brain excited by external impression on ye sentient extremities. Ergo a general view of ye N[ervous]. S[ystem]. and a particular description of its parts and their offices necessary to be prefixed to an account of ye functions – This ye reason of Cullen for beginning w[ith]. it.

But he went on to say that 'a description of ye moving organs is all that is absolutely requisite – It is therefore needless to introduce ye N[ervous]. S[ystem]. strictly so called.'[88]

Allen modified this position when he came to deliver his lectures. At the outset he distinguished the two vital properties which were the definitive characteristics of living bodies: muscular power, or irritability; and nervous power, or sensibility. These 'two leading characters', he argued, 'afford the foundation of an arrangement of the animal functions, which is perhaps the best that has hitherto been offered'.[89] Allen went on to discuss the various actions of the body as dependent on one or other of these properties. Consideration of the nervous system, as such, was left to the end of the course.

This demotion of the nervous system marked an important departure from the physiology of Whytt and Cullen; as Lawrence has remarked, eighteenth-century Scottish physiology was distinguished by 'its stress on the total integration of body function, the perceptive capacity or sensibility of the organism, and a preoccupation with the nervous system as the structural basis for these properties'.[90] In Allen this preoccupation with a central integrating organ had given way to a view of the body as decentralized but coherent. It would be easy to draw comparisons between this view of the body and a Whig social theory which refuses to acknowledge the predominance of any central power and diffuses authority throughout society – although Allen nowhere hints at such an analogy. The lectures embodied, however, a more complex set of political meanings.

Henry Brougham remarked that Allen 'had originally been a somewhat indiscriminate admirer of the French Revolution, and was not of the number of its eulogists whom the excesses of 1793 and 1794 alienated from its cause. Even the Directorial tyranny had not opened his eyes to the evils of its course'.[91] While he was no Bonapartist,[92] there is evidence that Allen never lost his enthusiasm for French republicanism. After the July Revolution of 1830 he wrote to Macvey Napier to celebrate 'the late brilliant events in France, and above all . . . the moderation of the Republican party, who have wisely given up the shadow to secure the substance [of the republic]'.[93]

During the 1790s Allen had carried this enthusiasm into his science. He placed great emphasis upon the significance for physiology of 'the present exalted & progressive Excellence' of chemistry.[94] In his lectures on respiration he declared:

> It is only since the brilliant discoveries of the french Chymists, who devoted their Labours to the elucidation of Phisiological phenomena, that any light has been thrown on this Subject[:] indeed the very purpose served by resp^{n} were [*sic*] till then unknown.[95]

In order to appreciate the full force of this assertion it is necessary to take account of the polemic *against* French chemistry that was waged in Edinburgh.[96] The rationalization of chemical terminology undertaken by the French was condemned by John Robison in 1803 as an aspect of the Jacobin mentality that had invented the Revolutionary calendar and introduced a new system of weights and measures.[97] Cockburn's dictum that 'everything' was soaked in the consequences of the French Revolution extended even to chemistry.

Allen's physiology also bore political meaning at a deeper level. His initial introduction of irritability and sensibility as the distinguishing principles of living bodies has a vitalist flavour. Elsewhere, he showed his opposition to any form of crude reductionism in physiology; Descartes' theory of secretion was, for example, dismissed as worthless.[98] Allen was firm that it was impossible to ascribe the phenomena of muscular irritability to the action of some simpler force:

> In mechanical arrangements, we lose in power what we gain in velocity; but this does not hold of musc^{r} contraction. – The prop^{y} by which musc^{r} fibres contract is one *sui generis*, and not capable of being resolved into any more general law of nature.[99]

Muscular action therefore differed from the motion of a machine because 'there is no production of Power in machines, but there is a Production of Power in muscles – hence it is a Simple power as gravity magnetism &c.'[100]

Allen was, however, equally critical of Stahl's animism and of similar attempts to explain phenomena by reference to an immaterial vital principle. 'The Stahlian Philosophers', he declared, 'accounted for Secretion by the influence of the soul, by a vis essentialis a "vita propria" a specific action &c. these terms equally vague & unsatisfactory are only Cloaks for ignorance –'.[101] He also attacked the more recent vitalist theories of the Viennese professor, Joseph Jacob Plenck (1738–1807). Plenck had argued that living solids and fluids possessed a vital principle 'which hinders them from obeying the laws of Chem^{l} Affinities, w^{h} they do when the Vital Principle has ceased'. This, Allen thought, was simply a refinement of John Hunter's theory of the life of the blood.[102]

He objected to Plenck's theory, and to George Fordyce's contention that digestion was effected by 'the *living power* of the Stom^{h}', because they suggested that the normal laws of chemistry were somehow suspended in the living body by the action of the vital principle. In fact, 'The more we know of the Animal Economy the less reason have we to suppose that other Chem^{l} agents are there employed, than in the rest of nature – indeed every investigation makes[?] in favour of the Contrary –'.[103] The assimilation of aliment into the blood, for example, 'is not so difficult to account for chem^{ly} as we might at first Sight imagine'. The blood and the alimentary matter 'consist of the same elementary Principles being diff^{tly} combined indeed & in very diff^{t} Proportions & . . . the Process tho. more complex indeed is nothing more than an ordinary Chemical experiment –'.[104]

Allen did not deny that chemical processes might take unique forms within the living body; but he maintained that in such instances attention should focus upon the peculiar circumstances that might be responsible. Thus in the case of absorption,

> may we not suppose that the Absorbent System acts very fully in producing these great Changes. that this System does not indiscriminately take up every fluid in w^{h} their mouths may be immersed but only such as by an unknown law they are fitted for. & it is very probable that they do this by a law very similar to chem^{l} affinity and this a variety of circumstances tend to prove -[105]

The presumption, therefore, had to be toward the validity of ordinary chemical principles in the explanation of physiological phenomena. Moreover, the doctrine of chemical affinity could be invoked to explain in a non-vitalistic way apparently purposive processes such as selective absorption. Chemistry in conjunction with anatomy was also the best hope for providing an adequate explanation of secretion.[106] Such insistence upon the uniform application of chemical laws to vital processes made possible a form of physiological determinism: 'The laws of chem^{l} affinity must in the same circ^{s} always and necessarily produce the same effects.'[107]

Allen thus denied the need to suppose some mysterious, immaterial agent in the body. Vital processes were all, at least in principle, explicable in terms of the laws of physical science; chemistry, in particular, offered rich promise to physiology. The alternative hypothesis of 'the influence of the vital principle over the chemical changes that take place in the body' was, in Allen's view, 'a matter of great obscurity'. It could imply, among other possibilities, that 'in addition to the chemical affinities there is also an unknown principle superior to and directing them'.[108]

The existence of this superior agent was, however, much insisted upon by some. The Edinburgh chemist, Thomas Thomson (1773-1852) in his *System of Chemistry* (1802) took a directly opposite view of digestion to that offered by Allen. 'What is the power', he asked,

> which prevents the gastric juice from acting on the stomach during life? Certainly neither a chemical nor mechanical agent, for these agents must still retain the same power after death. We must, then, of necessity, conclude, that there exists in the animal an agent very different from chemical and mechanical powers, since it controuls these powers according to its pleasure. These powers therefore in the living body are merely the servants of this superior agent, which directs them to accomplish always one particular end.[109]

Because of the action of this superior power, 'all the substances are not left at full liberty to obey the laws of their mutual affinities'. Thomson conceded, however, that the vital principle 'is not able to exercise an unlimited authority over the chemical powers; sometimes they are too strong for it'. When the animal died, 'the chemical and mechanical agents, which were formerly servants, usurp the supreme power, and soon decompose and destroy that very body which had been in a great measure reared by their means'.[110]

This difference over the adequacy of the chemical agents to explain vital processes needs to be placed in the context of wider conflicts. I have argued elsewhere that at the turn of the nineteenth century the question of whether life should be seen as immanent within the organism or as the result of some superior power was linked to current preoccupations with the nature of the moral and social order.[111] Thomas Thomson's language makes it clear that the *subordination* of the body to the vital principle was a cardinal point: it exercised *authority* over the body, preventing the constituent substances from exercising *full liberty*. The material part of the body was, moreover, incompetent to sustain life and organization in the absence of this power. These emphases correspond to a political theory concerned to demonstrate the necessity of hierarchy and of a supreme authority to the maintenance of society.

Allen, on the other hand, presented a view of the body as an autonomous mechanism, in which seemingly purposive operations could be ascribed to the workings of natural forces. The doctrine of chemical affinities served this mechanistic conception of the 'wisdom' of the body particularly well: as John Barclay remarked in 1797, 'chemistry . . . has been led to observe that particular salts show a preference for particular bodies, that there is in them an appearance of choice'. Where Barclay differed from Allen was in his refusal to accept that such a mechanism could give a complete account of the design apparent in the organism. Chemical agents, he declared,

> are neither almighty nor everywhere present; . . . in the internal organical economy of living bodies they act but a part; and . . . like the other agents in nature, they are obliged to confine their operations within those limits which the great Author of being has prescribed.[112]

In Allen's concept of the organism, however, God had no role. There were no spiritual agents at work; there was no insistence on the necessary subordination of the parts to some central power. The social theory which approximates most closely to this concept of the organism is that of political economy, where the market is assumed to possess an autogenous capacity to regulate supply and demand and where the proper role of the sovereign power was strictly circumscribed.[113] Dugald Stewart drew an explicit comparison between the animal and the political economy:

> in the political system, as well as in the animal body . . . there is a sort of *vis medicatrix*, which is sufficient for the cure of partial disorders; and in the one case, as well as in the other, the errors of human art are frequently corrected and concealed by the wisdom of nature.[114]

Thomas Thomson, in contrast, argued that in both health and disease the balance between supply and demand in the body could only be achieved through the constant supervision and incessant agency of the vital principle.[115]

Allen's deposition of the brain and nerves from the pre-eminent place they had occupied in earlier Scottish physiology can now be seen more clearly as an attempt to demonstrate the redundancy of central control.[116] The most extended programme of physiological research outlined in Allen's lectures involved, not the nervous system, but the self-regulating mechanisms that preserved a uniform temperature in animals.[117]

There is, however, one passage in a set of notes taken at Allen's lectures that seems to contradict this view of him as an exponent of an immanentist concept of life. When discussing Hartley's concept of 'automatic' motions, he is reported as saying that 'Automatic Motion can only be referred to the Will of the Deity we cannot otherwise explain them'.[118] This is the sole reference to the deity in Allen's physiology; it is also the only suggestion that vital processes might depend on some outside power. The observation appears in a note apparently taken from another student's record of the lectures.[119] Its authenticity may therefore be questioned. It is in any case entirely uncharacteristic of Allen's thought.

More typical is his discussion of generation. Allen reviewed the debate between preformationists and epigenesists and decided in favour of the latter. He noted Bonnet's contention that 'no chemical Union could produce, so wonderful, complicated & uniform a machine as an organized body'; but responded:

> the powers of nature are not to be measured by our Imagination – As all Anim^{ls} have the power of assimilating inorganized materials, into an organized part, why sh^{d} we deny that the whole body may become organized from original inorganized Particles?[120]

Allen therefore sided in the great eighteenth-century debate over generation with those who exalted the power and self-sufficiency of nature and against those who maintained that matter was incapable of bringing forth life without the intervention of the deity.[121]

In 1800 the first volume of Cuvier's *Leçons d'Anatomie Comparée* was published; within eighteen months Allen had produced an abridged translation dedicated 'To the Gentlemen Attending his lectures on the animal economy.' Allen was attracted to the work not for its anatomical or taxonomic content, but because the book 'appeared to the Translator to convey a more correct idea of the essential attributes of life, and to afford a more comprehensive view of the relations that subsist between the different functions of the Animal Economy, than any work which he had seen'.[122]

Part of the attraction of Cuvier's concept of life was that it was framed in terms acceptable to a disciple of David Hume. 'The idea of *Life*', Cuvier declared,

> is one of those vague and obscure ideas suggested in regular and corresponding trains. Though unable to discover the nature and the relation between these trains of phenomena, we are satisfied of its existence; and this is sufficient for us to class them together, and distinguish them by an appropriate term, which the vulgar mistake for the name of a particular Agent or Principle; whereas, it is merely a general expression for the phenomena, that suggested the formation of the term.[123]

Life was not an entity, but a chain or circle of phenomena. The living body was the focus for a process whereby life was continually preserved and recreated. Cuvier expressed this dynamic notion of the organism in a famous metaphor:

> Instead of an uninterrupted union in the same particles of living matter, we discover a continual circulation proceeding without interruption, and yet fixed down within certain limits. In this view of living bodies they may be compared to so many eddies or whirlpools, into which inanimate materials are continually drawn; where they are combined together in various forms, detained for a certain time, and applied to different uses; but from which they are at last thrown out, and restored to the laws of unorganized matter.[124]

As well as being dynamic, Cuvier's was a holistic concept of life. Parts separated from the body

> die speedily, because they contain not within themselves any principle of motion, and only participate in the general motion which is produced by their union into an organized whole; so that, to use the language of Kant, it depends on the living body as a whole, what mode of existence shall belong to its different parts; whereas, among unorganized bodies, the mode of existence depends solely upon itself.[125]

It is easy to see why Allen responded with such enthusiasm to Cuvier's ideas. They crystallized a view of the organism toward which he had himself approximated. The notion of life as process rather than principle; the idea of the body as an interdependent whole in which there was no predominant centre; the recognition that vital operations might be *both* subject to the same laws as inorganic matter and yet form a discrete realm of discourse: these were all intimated in Allen's lectures. Cuvier also articulated another of Allen's subtexts: the concept that function was, at least in principle, prior to structure, that physiology was not merely a form of *anatomia animata*. Allen therefore stands apart from much of early nineteenth-century British physiological discourse which continued to insist on a close alliance with anatomy.[126] John Barclay, for instance, in the article 'Physiology' in the 3rd edition of the *Encyclopaedia Britannica* insisted that 'Physiology in general and the study of anatomy are so closely connected, that, as Haller imagined, they can hardly be separated even in idea.'[127]

Conclusion

A year after the appearance of his translation of Cuvier, Allen left Edinburgh to join the Hollands on their tour of the continent. Here, his career as a man of science and medicine is usually supposed to end, and his endeavours as a man of letters to begin. The transition was not, however, quite so abrupt. While still in Edinburgh Allen already demonstrated some of the literary interests for which he was later noted. While attending Allen's physiology course, Francis Horner recorded a conversation in which

> Allen made an excellent observation to me . . . when I was mentioning to him my plans of historical reading: he proposed to divide history into its general events, and, before studying, *tout de suite*, the annals of the world in chronological order, to take those great events, one after the other, and investigate their several causes and various consequences.[128]

Moreover, although Allen abandoned the profession of medicine after settling in London, he did not entirely eschew its practice. On occasion he ministered to acquaintances who had been taken ill. When one of these offered him an ornate snuff box by way of thanks, Allen replied: 'When I gave up the practice of physick I formed a resolution, from which I have never departed, of not accepting, on any account whatever, of any remuneration . . . for such medical assistance as I might afterwards have an opportunity of rendering my friends'.[129]

In cases of serious illness in the Holland House circle, Allen acted as a medical manager marshalling advice from various practitioners as well as offering his own opinions. He was involved in the consultations in London and in Edinburgh concerning Francis Horner's condition.[130] When Georgina Fox, the Hollands' youngest child, fell ill in 1819, Allen was actively engaged in her treatment. He solicited opinions from, among others, John Thomson, and kept a detailed account of the case.[131] When the child eventually died, Matthew Baillie wrote to Allen urging the desirability of an autopsy.[132]

Allen also maintained an interest in medical politics. In April 1830 John William Turner sent him a copy of a petition protesting against a proposed tax upon licentiates of the Royal College of Surgeons of Edinburgh in the hope that Allen might be able to exert political influence against the measure.[133] Three years later Allen published his *Thoughts on Medical Reform*, a contribution to current debates on how to improve the structure and education of the medical profession. The time had arrived, he declared, 'when our medical, like our other estabishments, must undergo a thorough and complete revision'.[134] While scathing about the low quality of many Scottish medical graduates, he held that 'no public body has exerted itself more steadily and judiciously in improving the education of general practitioners than the Royal College of Surgeons at Edinburgh'. He therefore urged that the education of GPs nationally should be based on the model established by the Edinburgh surgeons.[135]

Allen was still seen as an authority on medical science after his removal from Edinburgh. Charles Bell in 1811 asked him for his opinion about the sketch of the Anatomy of the Brain I sent you. I mean to spend some of my last years on the investigation of the subject anatomically. I should like to be corrected before the long habit of thinking myself right shall have made me obstinate.[136]

The work in question was the *Idea of a New Anatomy of the Brain*, privately circulated among a select group, in which Bell argued that the anterior and posterior roots of the spinal cord possessed distinct functions.[137]

Allen also retained his interest in metaphysics. He corresponded on the subject with, among others, Dugald Stewart.[138] All these continuities with his Edinburgh career might, however, be considered as peripheral to Allen's main intellectual endeavours during his years in London. His principal writings were erudite discussions of constitutional history. These were not produced in a spirit of dispassionate scholarship, but as contributions to contemporary political debates; Allen stood in a long line of Whigs who looked to the ancient history of the constitution for resources with which to press their present claims.[139]

The most important of these works was the *Inquiry into the Growth of the Royal Prerogative in England*, first published in 1830. In his review of the book, Henry Brougham declared that, besides its scholarly merits, 'it possesses an additional title to the regards of those who love liberty, and value the institutions which are at once its best gift and its surest safeguards; it breathes throughout a warm love of freedom, and a firm spirit of resistance to slavish maxims'.[140] Allen's historical approach to constitutional problems showed the possibility of avoiding both the extremes of 'modern zealots for liberty and popular rights', on the one hand, and of Benthamite utilitarianism on the other.[141] But, most importantly, Allen's argument dealt a heavy blow to doctrines which located the source of sovereignty, not in the people, but in some transcendent authority.

He set out to undermine the doctrine that 'the legal authority of the king of England is absolute and irresistable, that he is the minister and substitute of the Deity; that all are under him while he is under none but God'.[142] Allen abhorred all the

> indecent attempts of churchmen to impress a character of divinity on Kings, to inculcate on their subjects the obligations of passive obedience and non-resistance as religious duties, to found their title on a delegation from heaven, and with impious flattery to exalt them above the Almighty, by maintaining, that the 'most high, sacred, and transcendent' of relations is the 'relation between King and subject.[143]

Such a notion of government was clearly incompatible with the Lockean doctrine that 'to obtain security for persons and property, was the great end for which men submitted to the restraints of civil government'.[144] The source of political authority, on this view, lay with the people, not with the deity.

In private Allen took a dim view of monarchy. As William IV neared death, Allen, in a letter to Macvey Napier, expressed his doubts of the ability of 'a girl of eighteen' to govern; 'what a strange institution is monarchy', he lamented, 'even when controlled by the long practice of an established Constitution!'[145] In public he was prepared to accept hereditary monarchy, but only if the constitutional role of the king was defined in Whig terms. The crown was not the personal property of the holder; it was 'an office or trust for the benefit of others; that if it has been made hereditary, it is only for the purposes of public utility'.[146]

He took special exception to any doctrine that might serve to sustain an alternative, transcendental, concept of kingship. In particular, he singled out the medieval concept that

> the King of England has in him two bodies or capacities; that he has a natural body, and a politic or mystical body; that his natural body is subject to the casualties and infirmities of other men, but that his body politic is utterly exempt from weakness and passion, secure alike from the helplessness of infancy and from the imbecility of age; that these two bodies, thus differently constituted, exist not apart, but are incorporated in one person; making one body, and not two bodies – corpus incorporatum in corpore naturali, et corpus naturale in corpore corporato – in such a manner that the politic body includes in it the natural body, and the natural body has in it the public body.[147]

Allen objected to this concept of kingship because it imparted a supernatural element to the monarch; implied that he possessed a wisdom above the merely human; and that the hereditary transmission of his office was something more than a socially useful expedient. On the basis of such mystical notions, 'many of the prerogatives of the real King have been surreptitiously introduced and established under the colours of his ideal prototype'.[148]

It is therefore possible to discern a unifying thread running through Allen's thought that spans the gulf opened by his abandonment of a medical career and departure from Edinburgh. In his 1790 dissertation to the Royal Medical Society he sought to explicate the workings of the human mind without any reference to an immaterial principle. In his lectures on physiology he constructed an account of vitality which dispensed with any form of superadded vital principle as the condition of life and organization. In his political writings, he propounded a naturalistic concept of monarchy which denied that any divine efflation was mingled with the corporeal reality of the king.

Allen himself felt, moreover, that he had never abandoned or compromised his early political ideals. Despite his long exile he retained a keen interest in Scottish affairs. When in 1833 Allen published a *Vindication of the Ancient Independence of Scotland* he exulted at what he saw as the ultimate triumph of the cause for which he had fought in the 1790s:

> After a struggle of forty years with a selfish, jobbing oligarchy, [the Scots] have obtained the same political rights as the people of England. That they have exercised the power committed to them with sense, calmness, and resolution, has been most gratifying to one who prides himself in being among the few unchanged survivors of those persecuted men who began the contest now so fortunately terminated in favour of the rights and liberties of his countrymen. To the Scottish nation he dedicates these pages in vindication of their ancient independence. May they never forget they inhabit the land 'where Wallace fought – where Buchanan wrote – and where Fletcher spoke'![149]

Allen's invocation on the eve of the Victorian era of such Old Whig icons as Buchanan and Fletcher is significant in defining his place in the history of political thought. He was perhaps the last term in a tradition of republican freethinkers that reached back to the seventeenth century.[150] As with such precursors as John Toland, Allen's ideas on society and nature need to be seen as aspects of a single endeavour.

3

The Old Chairmaker

And Thomson's wide and letter'd name,
For sense acute, and language strong:
And Barclay's great and learned fame,
Will bear their tide of strength along.[1]

Introduction

John Thomson's role in the cultural politics of late eighteenth-century Edinburgh has been described above. He is, however, better known for two other achievements. He was the author of a biography of William Cullen which has still not been superseded. Second, he showed a remarkable aptitude for creating academic positions for himself to fill. In the course of his career Thomson engineered the erection of no less than three professorships in Edinburgh: surgery (1804) at the Royal College of Surgeons, and military surgery (1806) and general pathology (1831) at the university. This talent did not meet with general approval: the *Lancet* remarked acidly that Thomson was 'said to have been the manufacturer of more chairs than would furnish a modern drawing-room'.[2]

The various aspects of Thomson's life should not, however, be considered in isolation. The different threads of his career were closely intertwined; in particular, his Whig politics had a major impact on his professional progress. This effect was mixed. At times Thomson's political persona and connections thwarted his ambitions; on other occasions they were crucial to his success.

It is useful to consider Thomson as a type of *entrepreneur*. The commodity in which he dealt was the kinds of medical knowledge for which there was a demand or for which a demand could be generated. He was far from unique in playing this role in the early nineteenth-century Edinburgh medical school. His success was, however, exceptional. Of the three chairs Thomson created two were short-lived. The chair of general pathology was to prove more durable; and Thomson did much to secure the institutional status of pathology in Britain. He contributed, moreover, to defining the *content* of pathological discourse: he did not deal merely in finished goods, but was actively engaged in the manufacture of new forms of medical knowledge. This aspect of his activity will be considered in the following chapter.

By about 1792–3 Thomson had decided upon a two-track approach to professional advancement. On the one hand, he sought to establish himself as a surgeon; on the other, he looked around for means to commence as a teacher. He thus confronted the opportunities and obstacles that faced any prospective medical teacher in Edinburgh at the turn of the nineteenth century. The most obvious course might seem to be to seek entry into the university medical school. The character of the Edinburgh professoriate, however, effectively eliminated this option.

Professors and patrons

The establishment of the Faculty of Medicine in Edinburgh University is usually dated to 1726. In that year four fellows of the Royal College of Physicians were appointed professors of medicine. By the end of the eighteenth century there were seven medical chairs in the university: anatomy, practice of medicine, institutes of medicine, chemistry, botany, midwifery and materia medica. The patronage of all these chairs bar one lay with the Town Council of Edinburgh.[3]

The Council enjoyed this role because Edinburgh University was originally a civic institution – it was the 'Town's College'.[4] As well as appointing professors the Town Council was responsible for the finance and general government of the university; they also claimed the right to regulate its academic programme. Although the professors strenuously resisted these pretensions in the early nineteenth century, the right of the Town Council to control virtually every aspect of university life was eventually affirmed by the Court of Session.[5]

The university was therefore almost entirely dependent for its personnel and constitution on the burgh government. The Town Council of Edinburgh consisted of 33 members: a provost, four baillies, a dean of guild, treasurer, three merchant councillors, two trades councillors, and six ordinary and eight extraordinary council deacons. The previous year's officers also continued to sit on the council. Much business was conducted not by the full council but by the 25 'ordinary' members. The affairs of the university were the responsibility of a special College Committee chaired by the Lord Provost. There was no trace of democracy in the way in which the Council was selected. As Hugh Arnot wrote,

> The town-council are not elected by suffrage of the householders at large, nor even by that of the burgesses. They are, in part, elected by the members of the fourteen incorporations, and they partly choose their own successors. The merchants have not, as merchants, any vote in electing the town-council; for the whole merchant guild is represented by the merchant members of the town-council for the time being. The grocers, printers, tallow-chandlers, barbers, vintners, and stablers, as such, can neither elect or be elected.[6]

In fact, only existing members of the Council enjoyed this suffrage: 'The principle of the closed shop and the self-perpetuation of power could hardly go further.'[7]

Despite these unpromising credentials, the Town Council in the eighteenth century generally distributed its academic patronage judiciously. Under the supervision of George Drummond capable teachers were appointed to vacant chairs enhancing the university's reputation and contributing to the prosperity of the city.[8] But after 1800 doubts were increasingly voiced about the competence and probity of the Town Council as a regulator of the university: R. Mudie declared that they were 'the most unfit patrons of a school of philosophy, or indeed of any thing learned or liberal, that human imagination could devise'.[9]

The Council was not, however, an autonomous agent; it was influenced in its decisions by various pressures. Under the Dundas regime the councillors enjoyed little freedom of choice being 'little else than a pair of bagpipes, upon which the said faction discourses whatsoever music it chooses'.[10] Candidates for chairs and their supporters accordingly addressed their pleas to members of the Dundas family. When in 1819 the Lord Provost of Glasgow wrote to Melville in favour of Robert Graham's candidature for the botany chair at Edinburgh, he acknowledged that 'This being a crown Appointment, your Lordship is considered to be an all powerful Influence.'[11] Given Dundas's influence over the Town Council, much the same could be said of all university appointments. Academic patronage therefore suffered from what Whigs saw as the general political corruption of the period.

The ruling faction included among its adherents, moreover, most of the university professors who, with few exceptions, were staunchly Tory. Although the professors had no formal role in making appointments, they were consequently able to exert some influence on the patrons by invoking the reciprocal obligations of party loyalty. This was done either directly by professors coming to an 'arrangement' with councillors or indirectly by lobbying Dundas or his subordinates. As a result, appointment policy reflected the concerns and prejudices of the professoriate.

If Thomson can be viewed as an entrepreneur in the market for medical knowledge, then the university professors can be regarded as a self-perpetuating cartel which jealously defended what they saw as their prerogatives. This was to a large extent an hereditary caste; when chairs fell vacant they were usually filled from within the ranks of the professoriate or simply bequeathed to relatives. It was extremely difficult for a rank outsider like Thomson to secure any of the existing chairs.

The professors were, moreover, resistant to any increase of their number by the creation of *new* chairs. Underlying this hostility to innovation was the view that the field of medical science was a finite asset susceptible of only strictly limited expansion. In the words of a memorandum from the Senatus Academicus to the Town Council of 1798, 'the multiplying of Professorships especially on new branches of Education whose importance is not obvious . . . does not promise to advance the prosperity or dignity of the University'.[12] Any increase in the number of teachers seeking to exploit this asset could only be achieved at the expense of the current tenants. There were sound economic grounds for this stance. The professors relied for most of their incomes on student fees; they supposed that any new chair could only be supported by drawing students away from existing courses.[13]

Usually the professors were successful in resisting proposals for expansion; numerous plans for new chairs in the later eighteenth and early nineteenth centuries were effectively scotched.[14] The medical professors were particularly vigorous in defending their rights; above all, the Monros were ever on guard against incursions upon their domain as professors of anatomy and surgery. These attitudes were perhaps most evident in 1816 when a proposal to create a new chair of comparative anatomy and veterinary medicine was entertained by the Town Council.

Comparative anatomy was a rising science in the early nineteenth century largely because of the achievements of Georges Cuvier in France. By coupling the subject with veterinary medicine members of the Council hoped to attract new students to Edinburgh; they pointed out that with the ending of the Napoleonic Wars there might otherwise be a diminution in enrolments.[15]

Contrary to the received view of the Town Council as composed of ignorant and unlettered men, the committee appointed to consider the proposal were remarkably enlightened and sophisticated in their endorsement of the proposal. They cited 'the splendid labours of *Cuvier*' in order to demonstrate the scientific importance of the subject.[16] They also suggested that

> An addition to our knowledge of the diseases of Animals might illustrate and generally contribute to our knowledge of the diseases of the human body, and the frequent opportunities of dissecting, and making experiments upon Animals, and the facility of conducting such enquiries would if well pursued, materially promote these

> objects. Physiology might likewise be expected to reap much advantage from such investigations[.][17]

The response of the learned professors to the proposal was in stark contrast to this liberal attitude. A committee of the Senatus Academicus reported that the creation of the new chair would be 'inexpedient'. They argued that while comparative anatomy was a true science, veterinary medicine was a mere art best left to empirics and farriers. Insofar as the subject was amenable to exposition in 'mere Academical Lectures', it was already taught in the university by the Professor of Agriculture. The committee also opposed the establishment of a veterinary hospital connected to the university. The professors were no less hostile to the creation of a chair devoted solely to comparative anatomy; such an institution would, they argued, be redundant:

> Although Comparative Anatomy forms no part of the Title of any existing Professorship of this University, and altho' it be not mentioned in any of the present Commissions, it is by no means overlooked in the actual Course of Instruction. In various points of view, it comes within the provinces of the several Professors of Anatomy, Physiology, Natural History and Agriculture, and even if a Chair were to be Established for the sole purpose of Teaching Comparative Anatomy, these Professors must be permitted to continue to Teach it[.]

The professors of anatomy, in particular, had, the report alleged, successfully taught the subject in the past, 'and the present Professor has been prevented only by his conviction of the little demand for Instruction in this branch of his Subject, from giving a separate Course of Lectures on Comparative Anatomy'.[18]

In a letter to the Lord Provost, Alexander Monro Secundus put the objections to the new chair more explicitly in terms of the proprietary interests of the existing professors. The 'appointment of a new Professor cannot fail to be a most direct interference with my province as well as with the provinces of Professors Coventry & Jameson'. Monro pointed out that professors had invested a great deal of time and money in their posts: 'If the intended plan were adopted, it is obvious, that after having done so, they are liable to intrusion by another person being appointed to teach the very same branch of Science.'[19]

Such opposition to curricular innovation militated against any prospective professor regardless of his politics. The intended incumbent of the new comparative anatomy chair was John Barclay, a loyal Tory. When, however, the aspirant academic was a member of the political opposition, the obstacles in his path became still more formidable.

The Dundas clan disposed of university appointments as part of the general patronage in their gift.[20] The same considerations applied in filling a chair as in appointing a postmaster or an excise officer. Supporters were to be rewarded; opponents were to be reminded of the folly of their ways. Lord Holland complained that 'In furthering the views of his friends, or thwarting those of his opponents, [Melville] was alike regardless of the interests of the Country. Patronage, thus employed, secured to him great authority in Scotland.'[21]

Candidates and their friends were well aware of the function patronage played within the Dundas economy of power. George Baird sought to reinforce Robert Christison's claims to the chair of medical jurisprudence by emphasizing

> the soundness of Dr Christisons *political* opinions & principles – and to *this* view of a Candidates character I cannot but believe that his Majestys Government will in every case be disposed to pay much attention – In an *University* it is of the last importance.[22]

Such considerations should indeed, James Finlayson argued, take precedence over the mere intellectual abilities of a candidate. When pressing the case that a cleric should be appointed to the vacant chair of rhetoric at Edinburgh, he argued that 'you can have much better security that both his political and religious principles are sound, than you can have for those of any mere *Philosoph* of the present days'. Finlayson was, in particular, concerned to eliminate the Whig Thomas Brown from the competition. He did not deny Brown's talents, but

> should feel myself disappointed if your Lordship should be induced to prefer a Young Man who has never had an opportunity of shewing any very strong attachment either to the Constitution or to the Religion of his Country, to Men who in other respects are his equals, and who can plead recommendations to the favour of Government which he wants.[23]

Discrimination against Whigs was especially apparent at Glasgow University. Francis Horner wrote to Jeffrey in 1806 that 'I hope your only reason for calling [Lockhart] Muirhead a Whig, is to establish him in my good Graces; for if he really is so, it will stand very much in his way. Let him conceal his liberality, till he gets his professorship'. Muirhead was a protégé of John Millar. His attempts to have his lectureship converted into a full chair had been thwarted because of his political principles; Charles Hope, the Lord Advocate, had sent a 'libel' against him to the Home Office which effectively precluded any appointment.[24] Similarly, when Richard Millar asked the Duke of Montrose why his lectureship in materia medica had not been converted into a chair, the Duke 'spoke handsomely of Dr Millar's talents and character, but added, that politics alone formed an insuperable bar to his promotion. Dr Millar had always been a Whig, and was regularly one of the Stewards to the Anniversary Fox dinner at Glasgow'.[25]

It was perilous therefore to be a Whig. There were, however, compensations. When a Whig ministry came to power there was a natural tendency to succour those who had suffered discrimination in the past. Millar's reward came in 1831 when finally 'the principles for which he had been excluded are those of the Government'.[26] There was more involved in such appointments than merely a desire to right past wrongs. Whig governments were no less politically minded than Tories when distributing patronage: Jeffrey recommended a Mr McFadane to be Keeper of the Minute Book of the Court of Session on the grounds that he was 'the individual whom most of our political friends consider as best entitled to that situation'.[27] John Millar had supplied a theoretical justification for such manoeuvres. Since the Glorious Revolution, he claimed, the 'friends of liberty' had been especially concerned to curtail a new threat to freedom: that posed by the crown's ability to place its partisans in position of influence throughout society by means of its patronage. Since the majority of the population tended to defer to the opinions of such placemen, whether they favoured the cause of freedom or of subordination, 'It is of . . . infinite consequence to have a number of partisans scattered through the nation, at all times zealous to support the administration, and ready to extol their measures.'[28] Even high-minded and philosophic Whigs were not, moreover, indifferent to the claims of friends and family; Jeffrey on one occasion solicited John Allen's assistance in an effort to obtain the Chair of Botany at Glasgow for his brother-in-law.[29]

University appointments did, however, possess a special significance for proponents of philosophic Whiggery that set them apart from other forms of patronage. The nascent liberalism of the late eighteenth century placed great stress upon the importance of 'opinion' in laying the foundations of a rational and just polity. Universities were seen as centres where the opinions of those who would in future wield political power could be shaped according to sound Whig principles. Millar and Dugald Stewart were outstanding examples of professors who set out quite deliberately, and with some success, to play this role of moral and political tutor.

The peculiar relationship of the Town Council to the university, the hostility of the professoriate to encroachments upon their domain, and the politicization of academic appointments were all to have a major influence upon John Thomson's attempts to establish himself as a medical teacher in Edinburgh. These efforts began, however, outwith the walls of the university.

Extramural teaching and the College of Surgeons

The university offered no immediate prospects for an aspirant medical lecturer like Thomson – although it did present a challenge. The Faculty of Medicine was not, however, coextensive with the Edinburgh medical school. Beyond the fortifications of the university flourished a band of private lecturers who also offered medical instruction to the student population of the city. This extramural school had its centre at Surgeon's Square in close proximity to both the university and the Royal Infirmary.

The private lecturers were able to operate because of the varied demands of, and the considerable flexibility enjoyed by, those who came to Edinburgh for some form of medical education. Students intending to take the MD did have to attend the lectures of the university professors; but they formed only a minority.[30] The rest were able to move between university and extramural lectures at will according to their tastes and intentions.

The position of the extramural school was further buttressed by the fact that the university was not the only institution in the city giving some form of medical qualification. The License of the Royal College of Surgeons (RCS) of Edinburgh was taken by far more students than the degree of the university; the College *did* allow students to count attendance on extramural lectures when applying for its diploma. The surgeons and barbers of Edinburgh had been erected into a corporation in 1505. From the time of their union with the apothecaries in 1657 the surgeons ceased to work as barbers; and by 1722 the surgeons and barbers were completely separate. In 1770 the corporation began to style itself the 'College of Surgeons'; and eight years later it obtained a royal charter. To mark this change of status the surgeons began to cultivate a new image of surgery as an intellectual profession rather than a mere handicraft. They also took it upon themselves to produce surgeons who lived up to this ideal; after 1770 the College aspired to a prominent role in the licensing and education of surgeons not only in Edinburgh but throughout the empire.[31]

In contrast to the rigid conservatism of the university, the surgeons at the turn of the nineteenth century showed themselves receptive to innovations in medical education.[32] The surgeons also compared favourably with the Royal College of Physicians of Edinburgh in this regard; the physicians were, in fact, precluded by their constitution from erecting a medical school in rivalry to the university. When in the 1840s Allen Thomson composed a note on the relative influence of the two Colleges on medical education in Edinburgh, he remarked that the physicians had not hitherto been 'connected with Medical education'; on the other hand, to the College of Surgeons the medical profession

> owes a long and deep debt of gratitude for its liberality in throwing into abeyance the exclusive privileges as to the practice of which it was

> legally possessed, for its unremitting and most successful efforts to maintain at a high standard the terms on which its diploma is granted, and not less for the disinterested devotion it has expended its funds in the collection of a magnificent and instructive museum of healthy and morbid anatomy and the liberality with which it has thrown this museum open to the public.[33]

In fact, the policy of the College of Surgeon was less altruistic than Thomson implied. Far from being disinterested in their promotion of medical education, the surgeons calculated that their corporate interests would be served by nurturing an image of themselves as a liberal and learned body.

The College was especially concerned to raise the standard of surgical teaching offered in Edinburgh. While acknowledged as an outstanding school of physic, Edinburgh was in the eighteenth century regarded as inferior to London and Paris as a surgical seminary. There was no separate chair of systematic surgery in the university until 1831. The professor of anatomy was supposed to satisfy the need for such instruction by means of a supplementary course of lectures on surgical operations. In 1777 the surgeons petitioned the crown for the creation of a new chair of surgery in the university. The initiative was, however, thwarted by the Senatus Academicus. To consolidate his position, Monro persuaded the Town Council to add the words 'and surgery' to his commission as Professor of Medicine and Anatomy.[34]

The College was more successful in its encouragement of instruction in clinical surgery. It endorsed the private lectures given by John Rae and James Russell in the Royal Infirmary. As noted above, Russell was in 1803 appointed Regius Professor of Clinical Surgery in the university; it took him ten years, however, to gain this appointment. He had presented a memorial in favour of a 'Clinical and Pathological' professorship of surgery in Edinburgh University to Robert Dundas in 1793. In this document Russell showed his awareness of the sensitivity of the Senatus Academicus to any proposal that might impinge upon their privileges. Clinical lectures on surgery he insisted 'do not in the least interfere with the medical clinical lectures heretofore delivered on cases on internal diseases'.[35] He also sought to reassure the Professor of Anatomy that *his* interests would not be damaged by arguing that:

> Medical clinical lectures have ever been regarded as a necessary & very usefull supplement to the general courses of lectures on the theory and practice of Medecine [*sic*] delivered from the chairs in this university. And it is clear that Chirurgical clinical lectures bear exactly the same relation to the general doctrines of Surgery. So that the course of lectures upon Anatomy & general Surgery given by Dr Monro will not be injured by any such supplemental establishment.[36]

While the supply of surgical teaching in Edinburgh was deficient at the beginning of the nineteenth century, the demand for such instruction was at an unprecedented level. Between 1793 and 1814 Britain was almost continuously at war. The armed forces of the country were vastly expanded – and with them the army and navy medical services.[37] Young men crowded Edinburgh seeking the qualifications that would give them entry to the lower ranks of the military medical service. At the same time those already appointed took the opportunity to seek further instruction that might help them gain promotion.[38] John Thomson exploited this state of affairs to launch his career as a medical teacher.

Thomson at first planned to teach anatomy. He proceeded in 1792 to London where he enrolled in John Hunter's school in Leicester Square with the aim of making use of the superior facilities for dissection in the metropolis to equip himself to give anatomical lectures. But Thomson soon abandoned this plan – partly because of the capital costs involved and 'partly in consequence of the high impression which he had formed of the abilities of Mr John Bell, who about that time entered on this department of instruction in Edinburgh'.[39] Bell was a redoubtable surgeon-anatomist who pioneered a new style of anatomy teaching during the 1790s.[40]

Instead Thomson turned to the less cultivated field of surgical education. He began to give systematic lectures on surgery in a private house soon after his appointment in 1800 as one of the surgeons-in-ordinary at the Royal Infirmary. At the same time he engaged in clinical teaching at the Infirmary in conjunction with James Russell.[41] On the strength of this association, Russell in December 1803 applied to the Home Office for Thomson to be named conjoint professor of clinical surgery; nothing, however, came of the proposal.[42]

The resumption of war with France highlighted the potential importance of the military as patrons of medical education. The impact of the war on Edinburgh society as well as on the physical fabric of the city was considerable. The east coast of Scotland was regarded as a possible invasion site; and troops were also needed to put down any popular unrest. As well as the regular troops, volunteer regiments were raised and a militia recruited. The medical establishment was correspondingly increased and a military hospital established at the castle.

These developments prompted Thomson to militarize his teaching. Encouraged by Lauderdale's brother General Sir Thomas Maitland, he decided in the winter of 1803–4 to give a course of lectures on military medicine and surgery. He had no personal experience of these topics, but studied the best continental and British texts on the subject.[43] The course appears to have been a success: Francis Horner wrote to Thomson in January 1804 'I was happy to learn from Dr Jones, that you are lecturing to great effect'.[44]

Shrewd self-interest, as well as patriotism, motivated Thomson's decision to seek to make himself serviceable to the military:

> The idea of giving a course of military surgery he was the more readily induced to adopt, partly . . . by the circumstances of the times, and partly by his knowledge that the army and navy during the impending momentous conflict, must in great measure be supplied with surgical officers from among the young men educated in the medical school of Edinburgh, who, from the narrowness of their circumstances, could not afford to attend the hospitals in London, but must go immediately from the Edinburgh school into actual practice.[45]

A course on military surgery would therefore have a guaranteed audience. Moreover, by orientating his teaching so as to satisfy this demand, Thomson could hope to attract the favourable attention of the military authorities. Throughout his early career he sedulously cultivated this source of patronage.

In the summer of 1804 Thomson gave a further course on military surgery; he taught three times a week between May and August in the same room at the south-west of Surgeon's Square where John Allen lectured on the animal oeconomy. The contents of the course were, in part, what one would expect in a set of lectures directed at actual or prospective military surgeons: it included such topics as

> Incised Wounds, or Wounds inflicted by the Broad Sword or *Sabre* – Of Punctured Wounds, or Wounds inflicted by the Bayonet – Of Lacerated and Contused Wounds, or Wounds inflicted by Splinters of Wood, Pieces of Earth or Stone, Spent Balls, &c. &c. – Of Gunshot Wounds – Of the external Applications to be used in the different Kinds of Wounds, with the Mode of Dressing and Bandaging them.

The course was not, however, confined to such obvious matters. Thomson declared that

> In the conduct of this Course, the Attention of the Student will be particularly directed to the Pathology of the different injuries; and to the Reasons for which Operations or Medicines, recommended in the Treatment of them are to be employed.[46]

A strong theoretical element is thus apparent in Thomson's teaching from an early date; he stressed in particular the importance of a knowledge of pathological principles to rational surgical practice.

By the autumn of 1804 Thomson had delivered two courses on military surgery in the extramural school in addition to his previous lectures on the principles and practice of surgery and clinical teaching. According to his biographer,

> The beneficial influence of these courses was very speedily perceived by those interested in the improvement of surgical education in Edinburgh, and by none more promptly than by Mr Benjamin Bell and Mr Andrew Wood; and they revived a wish that had repeatedly been expressed in the College of Surgeons, to have the teaching of Surgery placed in this city upon a permanent and respectable footing.[47]

A faction within the College of Surgeons thus saw in John Thomson's teaching an opportunity to revive the old demand for a Professor of Surgery in Edinburgh. But instead of the previous notion that this chair should be located in the university, the proposal that now emerged called for it to be sited in the College of Surgeons itself.

Thomson's biography records that shortly before the commencement of the 1804-5 session a memorial was presented to the College signed by several fellows proposing his appointment as professor of surgery. What the biographer did *not* point out was that Thomson had himself written to these surgeons soliciting their aid in obtaining an appointment as 'Lecturer on Surgery' within the College.[48] The memorial dated 21 September 1804 was signed by Bell, Wood, and seven other fellows of the Royal College of Surgeons. They pointed out the inadequacy of the surgical instruction offered by the university, noting that one consequence of teaching the subject merely as an appendage to the anatomy course was that 'the attention of the Student will be directed to the performance of operations and but little if at all, to what must ever in practice constitute the principal part of his duty, namely the Medical treatment of Chirurgical diseases'.[49]

The memorial was approved by the College on 28 September and a committee established to draw up regulations for the new post. At this stage Andrew Wood

> stated that from his knowledge of Mr John Thomson one of their number and of the pains which he had taken to qualify himself for teaching Surgery he begged leave to propose him as a fit person to fill the office now established by the Royal College with the Title of Professor of Surgery of the Royal College of Surgeons.[50]

On 5 October the College ratified this appointment, leaving the question of Thomson's title open. John Bennet, one of the fellows, however, objected on the grounds that

> I consider such an election as giving an undue superiority and advantage to the Individual Member so elected; and operating to the evident prejudice of those members of the Royal College, who at present give or may afterwards wish to begin private lectures on Surgery.

Bennet also hinted at the opposition this new institution might arouse when he added 'I am tired of Law Suits, in which the Royal College has been lately too much engaged.'[51]

The committee set up to consider the terms of the appointment also anticipated an adverse reaction from other interests within the city. Thomson's title, in particular, might prove contentious: the designation 'Professor' could be seen as an encroachment on the prerogatives of the university and might 'meet with opposition from the Town Council of Edinburgh'. The committee maintained, however, that the College was fully within its rights to appoint a professor to teach its own mystery.[52] In an attempt to avoid conflict with the medical faculty they did stipulate that the hours of Thomson's lectures should not clash with the medical, clinical and anatomical lectures offered by the university.[53] The College agreed to advertise Thomson's new course in the Edinburgh, London, Dublin and Glasgow newspapers.

It was this advertisement that first alerted the Senatus Academicus to the College's initiative. The Principal presented the text of a letter of protest to the Lord Provost which declared that 'This procedure on the part of the College of Surgeons appears to several Members of the Senatus Academicus to be a direct violation of the Rights and Privileges of the Patrons, as well as to threaten, in its principle & its probable consequences, serious injury to the interests of the University.'[54]

The Town Council needed little prompting. On 31 October it put the RCS 'upon their Guard in relation to their late resolutions' regarding the chair. The Council warned the surgeons that

> it is their Intention to investigate this Subject, with the most minute and scrupulous attention, in order to ascertain the relative Rights of themselves as the head of this Community, and as Patrons of the University, as well as the Rights of the Royal College of Surgeons; and from the Result of that Investigation, to determine what steps shall be pursued in future.[55]

The Council sought also to put pressure on Thomson himself: on the morning that he was to deliver his first lecture,

> he received a letter from the Lord Provost . . . expressing a hope that he would not persevere in his intention of lecturing as Professor of Surgery, otherwise the Magistrates and Council would feel it to be their duty to interrupt him and dismiss his audience.

This threat was, however, subsequently withdrawn.[56]

The Town Council also asked the Lord Advocate 'to use your influence with His Majestys Ministers not to grant any Confirmation of or sanction to the

Measures taken by the Royal College of Surgeons, until the Rights of the respective bodys shall be ascertained, or until the Patrons of the College of Edinburgh be heard for their Interest'.[57] They were especially concerned that the War Office should in no way endorse the new chair. Charles Hope was happy to grant the Council's request; he sent the Lord Provost's letter to William Dundas, the Secretary at War, with a covering note:

> The inclosed speaks for itself – The Surgeons appear to be corporately & collectively mad – I send the letter to you rather than directly to the Secretary of State, because it is said to be a part of their plan to obtain some appointment & Establishment from the War Office, under pretence of instructing Surgeon's Mates –
>
> Therefore, show the letter to Lord Hawkesbury, & lodge the necessary Caveats in His & your own Offices, & any other, if other be necessary.[58]

The RCS had indeed sought to attract the support and approval of the armed forces. They announced in the advertisement promulgated on 5 October 1804 that 'Officers of the Medical Staff of the Army, and Surgeons and Surgeons' Mates of the Navy . . . will be entitled to attend these Lectures gratis.'[59] Thomson himself forwarded a copy of this extract to the relevant authorities. He also appealed to the military medical department's desire to improve the educational acquirements of candidates for its service, arguing that by 'extending the Course which has been intrusted to me by the College, to a period of six months, I hope . . . in some measure to rescue Surgery in this School from the imputation of being merely a manual art'. Thomson added that

> it would assist me greatly in the execution of these purposes could I obtain from the Medical Board a simple recommendation to the Gentlemen studying Medicine at this University & who may intend to enter afterwards into the service of the Army to attend my Lectures.

Such a recommendation 'could not fail of being immediately of material advantage to me'.[60]

The Army Medical Board considered this communication on 3 December and in reply sent a letter 'expressive of approbating and shall be ready to give the plan every support & countenance'.[61] At their quarterly meeting in November 1805 the RCS was able to record with satisfaction that the new chair 'has met with the fullest approbation of the Army Medical Board & of the Board of Sick & Wounded Seamen'.[62] Hope's efforts to sabotage the surgeons' attempt to obtain official sanction had failed; one advantage of the military medical establishment as a patron was the evident independence from the pervasive influence of the Dundas faction that they enjoyed.

After their initial belligerent noises the Town Council let the matter of the chair of surgery drop. Following representations from Benjamin Bell, the Lord Provost declined to join George Baird in an application to the government for the abolition of Thomson's chair.[63] The university, however, continued to pursue the matter during 1805. In January they received advice from the law faculty that there was little legal basis for the university's objections, and that it was inadvisable to take the issue to court. The report added that

> independent of the chances of Success, the expediency of stirring the Investigation is much to be called in question, as any Opposition given to the recent Institution of the Surgeons would tend strongly to bring it forward to public notice, and bestow upon it a degree of importance which, if left to itself, it never would, in all probability attain.

None the less, the Senatus Academicus decided in June to seek further legal advice.[64] Eventually, however, even the professors were forced to admit defeat.

Thomson held the chair of surgery at the Royal College of Surgeons for seventeen years. During that time he developed a distinctive concept of the scope and goals of surgical education: he sought to educate 'scientific' surgeons rather than to train skilful operators. The content of his lectures is considered more fully in chapter 4. Within two years of his appointment at the RCS Thomson had, however, achieved a still more notable coup by breaching the defences of the university itself.

Military surgery

The professoriate's automatic resistance to any attempt to add to their numbers made the creation of any new chair through Town Council patronage virtually impossible. Despite the Lord Provost's enthusiasm for the scheme, the proposal for a chair of comparative anatomy and veterinary medicine failed because of the opposition of the medical faculty. There was, however, an alternative route to academic innovation: the crown had the power to appoint Regius professors at Edinburgh as at all British universities. In Glasgow most of the medical chairs were crown appointments.

But in practice the Senatus Academicus and Town Council had a say even in such appointments. Thus James Russell's memorial in favour of a chair of clinical surgery was considered by a committee of the Senatus Academicus, which finally agreed to the proposal but only after imposing strict conditions to ensure 'the security of the Professor of Medicine, Anatomy & Surgery in the full enjoyment of his present rights'. Above all,

Russell's commission prohibited him from teaching a course on the practice of surgery from the new chair.[65]

This professorial veto could only be overcome when there was a will to do so at the centre of government. Conversely, no candidate could succeed if he was politically obnoxious to those in power. When Russell suggested that Thomson be appointed conjoint professor of clinical medicine, the Home Secretary scribbled on the reverse of the proposal: 'Is there any objection to it?'[66] Since the appointment did not take place we can infer that there *was* some insuperable objection, the nature of which became clear subsequently when it emerged that

> a *caveat* against Mr Thomson's receiving any appointment from the Crown had been lodged in [the Home] office for a considerable time; and that it had, on a previous occasion, prevented his receiving an appointment of a different sort, even after it had been promised him by two different ministers.

The reason for this proscription was that 'an impression has prevailed in some quarters, that Mr Thomson, at an early period of his medical career, took a share in political movements of a character hazardous to public tranquility, and particularly that he was a member of the association known under the name of the Friends of the People'.[67]

Thomson's biographer refuted this specific allegation. There was, however, no denying that Thomson was an ardent Whig; and this alone was enough to incur the displeasure of the party that held power during most of the first three decades of the nineteenth century. But in 1806 a narrow window of opportunity opened: the 'Ministry of All the Talents' led by Charles James Fox took office. Suddenly Thomson's political friends were the government.

Some of the Whig party were well aware that this was merely a temporary departure from the normal run of political fortunes; it was consequently imperative to make the best use of this brief interlude of power. The distribution of patronage was regarded as a key issue. Since the suppression in the 1720s of the office of Secretary of State for Scotland, Scottish business was discharged by local magnates who had the favour of the regime in London. Originally, Thomson's old benefactor Lord Lauderdale was to have control of Scottish affairs. However, because of a counter-claim from the Earl of Moira, no 'Scottish minister' was appointed; patronage in Scotland was instead confided to the Home Secretary.[68]

Francis Horner regarded Moira's bid as an attempt by 'the Dundasses & Hopes' to 'retain [the Scots] under the old disgraceful and illiberal system of management'. In words reminiscent of John Millar he set out the issues at stake:

> You must see at a glance what a crisis this is in the politics of Scotland; upon the settlement of this point it will wholly depend, whether it is possible so to embody the independent opinions of that part of the country as to give us a barrier, when the Whigs are again out of place, against the illiterate jobbing cabal by which we have been so vulgarly misgoverned for the last twenty years. The Whigs, believe me, will very soon be restored to their natural state of opposition to the Court.[69]

Whigs already holding university posts were given official recognition: Dugald Stewart was awarded a highly controversial sinecure. There was also an attempt to increase Whig representation in the Scottish universities. Lockhart Muirhead was at last promoted to a chair of natural history at Glasgow.

Thomas Thomson's account of this appointment and of its aftermath shows how Muirhead's elevation affected the political balance of the university. 'In the year 1807', Thomson recalled,

> Dr Lockhart Muirhead was appointed Regius Professor of Natural History, during the short Whig administration, after the death of Mr Pitt. . . . At that time political parties ran very high in the University, and they were very nearly matched, eight of the Professors being Tories, and six Whigs. Dr Muirhead was known to be a Whig. It became, therefore, an object with the Tories to prevent him, if possible, from having a vote at their elections. As the College is totally dependent on the Crown for its revenues, no step could have been taken, had not the sudden change of administration deprived all the political friends of Dr Muirhead of their influence.[70]

John Thomson's appointment as Regius Professor of Military Surgery in May 1806 therefore possessed a decided political significance. To his enemies it was another flagrant attempt by the Whigs to increase their academic representation. The manoeuvres to secure the chair began soon after the Whigs came to power. On this as on other occasions John Allen's position near the centre of political affairs was of service to his Edinburgh associates. When Allen intimated to Thomson that the opposition of the professors might prove a stumbling-block to any new Regius chair, Thomson looked to Dugald Stewart to give an *ex cathedra* judgement on the question. Stewart replied on 20 February:

> In consequence of the letter you showed me from Mr Allen, I have conversed with my friend Mr Dalzel, and we agree in thinking, that no reference to the Senatus Academicus is necessary in the erection of a new Regius Professorship. At least, to the best of our recollection no such reference was made when the Professorship of Practical Astronomy and of Natural History were established, altho. both of

> these might be considered as encroachments in some degree on College offices previously existing[.][71]

Armed with such assurances and encouraged by Lauderdale, Thomson proceeded to London in April to press his case in person. He was shrewd to call for a chair specifically of *military* surgery. In time of war this could be presented as a patriotic measure likely to contribute to the efficiency of the armed forces and the welfare of the troops. This was also an aspect of surgery which the Professor of Anatomy could not claim to encompass in his lectures, making it more difficult for Monro to send up the old cry of 'encroachment'. The need for some kind of academic institution for the education of military surgeons had, moreover, been canvassed by others.

John Bell in 1800 lamented that 'No plan of national education has ever been proposed. Every other branch of our profession is taught, apart and carefully, while Military Surgery, the most peculiar of all departments, has been left to chance.'[72] Bell stressed the value to the state of

> a body of well-educated men, thoroughly instructed not only in surgery, but in military surgery; not only in the cure and prevention of diseases, but in the cure and prevention of the diseases peculiar to those climates which are most destructive to our soldiers and sailors[.][73]

He called for the foundation of a School of Military Surgery devoted to the education of such men. The school would employ a professor who would teach the essentials of military surgery and medicine.[74] Thomson's proposed chair of military surgery can be seen as a more modest version of Bell's proposal. There are many similarities between the duties of Bell's hypothetical professor and what Thomson did in fact teach; in particular, he took on board Bell's notion that a professor of military surgery must also teach military *medicine*.

The issuing of Thomson's commission in May 1806[75] could, therefore, be justified in terms of the public interest. It might, however, also be seen as a reward for political services rendered. In January Henry Petty-Fitzmaurice – the future 3rd Marquess of Lansdowne – stood as Whig candidate for the Cambridge University seat. Francis Horner acted as Petty's election agent and sought support from among Cambridge graduates who also had Edinburgh connections. Horner advised a lieutenant that 'John Thomson will be best able to assist you in making out a list of names'.[76] Petty was elected and served as Chancellor of the Exchequer in the Whig ministry.

The university's reaction to Thomson's appointment was predictable. The affair of the RCS chair clearly still rankled; the Senatus Academicus insisted that

> the University, in receiving Mr Thomson's Commission do not mean to resign or renounce their right to take all competent & lawful measures which they may deem advisable for preventing Mr Thomson from holding his present Lectureship in Surgery under the College of Surgeons.

Most aggrieved were the Monros who protested that the military surgery chair 'truly and substantially, is an encroachment on our right & Franchise under our previous Commission as professors of medicine, Anatomy & Surgery'. They concluded that the government had been seriously misled. Despite these complaints, 'Mr Thomson being present was received & welcomed by the Senatus Academicus in the usual manner.'[77]

Thomson held the military surgery chair until 1822. He used the position to strengthen his links with the military establishment. He sought and eventually obtained an appointment to the military hospitals in Edinburgh. In 1811 he had petitioned the principal medical officers of the army for the right to conduct clinical teaching in these hospitals.[78]

In 1815 Thomson travelled to Brussels and helped tend the soldiers wounded at Waterloo. He regarded this as 'the greatest opportunity I have ever had of learning military surgery. And I will do all I can to avail myself of it.'[79] It was also an opportunity to impress the Army Board with his devotion to their interests. In recognition of these services he was appointed a staff surgeon to the army. Thomson was eager for the regular source of income such a post would bring; he wrote to his wife from Brussels that 'I should like much to get something permanent that we might sink it as we did the other military salary for the children.'[80]

He was, moreover, now able to proceed with his plan to give clinical lectures in the army hospitals. He also used the military depot hospital at the castle for research purposes, experimenting with new treatments in a way that would have impossible in private practice.[81] Thomson's links with the military thus supplied the lack of access to hospital patients from which he had suffered since his resignation from the Royal Infirmary in 1809.

Thomson's appointment as staff surgeon caused considerable resentment among long-serving military doctors. The fact that he continued to receive a full salary when others were reduced to half pay caused special bitterness. One officer sent a scurrilous letter anonymously to the War Office calling for Thomson's dismissal. Among the allegations was the claim that 'during the short Administration in 1806–7 some of his early Patrons who had the ear of Mr Fox got the Professorship [of Military Surgery] made for him'.[82]

The vigour of Thomson's response to these attacks is an indication of the importance he attached to his post as staff surgeon. His principal defence was his record as a teacher of surgery: he pointed out that

> in the winter session 1815–16, I gave admission without fee to my Lectures upon the Principles and Practice of Surgery to eighteen Medical Officers belonging to the army and to 62 Medical officers belonging to the Navy and that in the Summer Session of 1816 I delivered a course of lectures on Military Surgery which was attended by 110 students without fee of which 17 belonged to the Army and 28 to the Navy, and that this winter I have given out 51 gratis tickets for each of my courses of Lectures to Medical officers of the Army and 53 to those of the Navy.

Thomson also drew attention to the clinical teaching he had performed at the depot hospital for the benefit of the attending medical officers.[83]

By the early 1820s the link with the military hospitals had, indeed, become Thomson's chief incentive for persevering with his surgical teaching. He now had a substantial income from private practice to which courses attended largely by students who paid no fee could add little. When in 1822 as a result of a reduction in the military establishment he lost his position as staff surgeon he resigned the professorship of military surgery; he had relinquished his post at the RCS the previous year. Thomson had not, however, abandoned his academic ambitions, but merely redefined them.

The theory and practice of medicine

Between 1806 and 1820 John Thomson transformed his professional identity. From being a surgeon and professor of surgery he became a physician and teacher of medicine. Thomson charted the steps of this transformation in a pamphlet of 1824 when he described himself as one 'who has passed through the several graduations of Surgeon's apprentice; Apothecary's assistant, Surgeon's and Physician's clerk in a public Hospital; Surgeon-apothecary, or Family Practitioner; Doctor of Medicine; and who . . . is at length a Consulting Physician'.[84]

It is important to stress the continuous, non-saltatory, nature of this transition. This reflected the general fluidity of roles in the early nineteenth-century Edinburgh medical profession. The formal distinction between surgery and physic had never in practice been observed. The President of the RCS informed Melville in 1825 that 'The College of Surgeons of Edinburgh are in fact *Surgeon Apothecaries* – . . . and they continue to practice *Surgery* and *Pharmacy*'.[85] Most Edinburgh surgeons were, in effect, general practitioners. Conversely, an Edinburgh MD like Robert Christison, who had no formal surgical qualifications, performed 'the minor operations of Surgery just as well as I do strict Physic'.[86] Such versatility was, John Bell maintained, especially necessary to the military surgeon – 'accustomed to be at once physician, surgeon, and apothecary, to a number of men in seasons of infection and danger!'[87]

Thomson planned his teaching at the RCS and as Professor of Military Surgery at the university with an eye to the future requirements of his students. According to one of his auditors,

> the course of lectures delivered by Dr Thomson was valuable, not simply as a body of chirurgical instruction. From the method of arrangement which he adopted, and the subjects of which he treated, it followed that much information on medical pathology was communicated . . . . From these circumstances it resulted that the course of Dr Thomson, indispensable to the well-educated surgeon, was not less necessary to the physician; and hence there were few physicians at that time educated in Edinburgh who did not feel the importance of attending these lectures with the utmost regularity.[88]

One result of the comprehensive character of Thomson's courses was that his teaching had a protean aspect. Although formally part of surgical education, his lectures could easily be turned into instruction in the practice of medicine or in general pathology.

As early as 1808 Thomson began the process of redefining himself as a physician: in that year he obtained an MD from King's College, Aberdeen. In Februaryruary 1815, he became a licentiate of the Royal College of Physicians of Edinburgh. By this time, he was already practising as a consulting physician. A number of motives can be suggested for this shift. In the first place, Thomson was not an accomplished operative surgeon in the mould ofJohn Bell or Robert Liston; indeed, he resigned his surgeoncy at the Royal Infirmary after Bell publicly charged him with incompetence.[89] Also significant were the implications of Thomson's persona as a practitioner for his academic career. There was a change in the medical marketplace after 1815: with the cessation of hostilities, the demands of prospective military surgeons became a less important consideration. There were, moreover, severe limitations to the potential of surgery to serve as a vehicle for Thomson's developing ambitions.

He was dissatisfied with both his post at the RCS and with his university chair. Some time after 1815 Thomson drafted a memorandum outlining the case for a chair of surgery in the university. After outlining the deficiencies of the present mode of teaching surgery as an adjunct to the anatomy course, he went on to insist that 'The want of such a Professorship is not and cannot be supplied by the Professor of Clinical or Military Surgery as these Professors are prohibited by their Commissions from teaching the Principles and Practice of Surgery and have neither of them a place in the Medical Faculty'.[90] He pointed to the precedent of the University of Glasgow where the crown had endowed a Regius professorship of surgery.

Such pleas were, however, futile. The Monros were more than ever determined to defend their territory and possessed the political influence to do so successfully. In 1807 and 1808 Monro secundus petitioned Melville and his son for the defence of his rights. He complained that

> Two other Professors upon Surgery have within these few years, been appointed by His Majesty, in this University; One of whom is Entitled Professor of Clinical Surgery, the other Professor of Military Surgery, both of whom have received Salarys from his Majesty: and both of them encroach upon the Emoluments of that Department which I held, and now hold in Conjunction with my Son.[91]

Given this sense of grievance, Monro was not likely to countenance Thomson's proposal that the teaching of surgery should be entirely divorced from the patrimony of his chair and transferred to yet another new professor.

Thomson hinted at why his present position was unsatisfactory to him when he complained that the Professor of Military Surgery had 'no place in the medical faculty'. Regius professors in the University of Edinburgh were excluded from some of the most important and lucrative prerogatives available to their colleagues: they could not examine candidates for the MD degree; and they were denied the right to give clinical lectures in the Royal Infirmary. These privileges were reserved to holders of Town Council chairs who had the words 'of medicine' in their commissions. Thus Monro, for example, was 'Professor of Medicine and Anatomy' and therefore entitled both to examine and to act as a clinical professor. Thomson coveted these rights; he was, in particular, anxious to obtain the access to hospital patients that clinical lectures would give.

Regius professorships were also defective in another crucial respect. Because they were in the gift of the crown it was difficult to establish any hereditary rights in them. By the 1820s Thomson had conceived the ambition of founding a medical dynasty. The desideratum therefore became a professorship that gave access to the Faculty of Medicine and which Thomson could hope to pass on to his son

Thomson's initial strategy was to seek one of the existing medical chairs. In 1819 the Chair of Botany became vacant upon the death of Daniel Rutherford. The post attracted Thomson's attention because the full title of the chair was that of Professor of *Medicine* and Botany; its holder consequently enjoyed the full rights of a member of the medical faculty. Thomson offered himself for this position even though he had no obvious qualifications as a botanist. At the same time he suggested that

> in the event of the patrons wishing to secure for the chair of botany the services of a distinguished cultivator of that branch of science, not belonging to the medical profession, – its medical duties, including that of delivering clinical lectures in medicine, might advantageously

> be transferred to a chair of surgery, for which, in the event of its being created, he purposed to be a candidate.[92]

He may have learned that the Senatus Academicus hoped to attract the distinguished London botanist Robert Brown to Edinburgh;[93] by suggesting a way in which the clinical could be divorced from the scientific aspects of the chair Thomson obviated one objection to this appointment.

In the event both the professors and Thomson were disappointed: Melville awarded the chair to Robert Graham who had the support of politically powerful patrons, notably the Lord Provost of Glasgow.[94] Graham and his supporters laid stress upon his experience as a physician and clinical teacher when outlining his qualifications.[95] The manner of Graham's appointment caused outrage in Edinburgh. *The Scotsman* described it as 'one of the grossest insults ever offered to the public'. The paper complained that not even the Town Council had been consulted, although they were nominally joint patrons of the chair. The 'interests of science' and the public good had been sacrificed to the gratification of private interest.[96]

In the spring of 1821 a still more attractive opening occurred when James Gregory, the Professor of the Practice of Medicine, died.[97] Thomson published a formidable set of testimonials in his favour.[98] In the printed announcement of his candidacy he declared that

> to obtain the honour of the appointment I now solicit, has long been the highest object of my ambition; and that the hope I might one day be considered as qualified to teach the Practice of Physic, has been the guide of my general studies, and the principle which has animated my labours in the acquisition and communication of medical and surgical knowledge.[99]

As well as these public measures Thomson sought the support of his political friends. John Allen solicited further letters from, among others, his former student George Birkbeck.[100] Lauderdale was also approached; while willing to help he was, however, pessimistic about the value of his patronage: 'I confess as far as I can judge my writing such a letter as [Thomson] mentions to the Provost would not be advantageous for him and certainly not likely to do away any prejudice against him on the score of politicks.'[101] Thomson's carefully cultivated association with the military did, however, yield a still more eminent patron. At the behest of the Army Medical Department the Duke of York declared:

> I am assured that Dr Thompson [*sic*] is eminently qualified for the practice Chair; and that there is no individual more proper to succeed those valuable Men, Cullen and Gregory, or who is more able

> to uphold the distinguished respect which the University of Edinburgh has enjoyed.[102]

It was all to no avail. When the Town Council first considered the vacancy they made a show of declaring their impartiality between the candidates. *The Scotsman* welcomed these protestations, arguing that for the good of the university the chair must be bestowed upon the individual 'who has given the highest proofs of skill and proficiency in the science of medicine' – and not on the basis of politics or candidates' connections. But they added: 'knowing what the system is, we expect nothing disinterested or patriotic to be done under it'.[103]

These fears proved well founded; despite their declared impartiality and autonomy the majority of the Town Council were content to acquiesce in the traditional '*system* of private arrangement, and *routine* promotion'.[104] In other words they bowed to pressure from the professors to appoint an internal candidate: James Home was promoted from the chair of materia medica to become the new professor of the practice of physic.

Anticipating defeat Thomson withdrew from the contest before the vote was taken. In his letter to the Town Council he regretted that 'an *arrangement* had been formed which would *necessarily preclude competition*'.[105] The full ramifications of this 'arrangement' emerged later: the professors had evidently agreed among themselves that upon Home's promotion Andrew Duncan junior would move to the materia medica chair, while William Pulteney Alison became the new professor of the institutes of medicine. Thomson applied for the latter position, but was defeated by nine votes to nineteen. After this third rebuff he denounced the corruption of the prevalent system in a letter to his supporters on the Town Council; he had

> felt the same reluctance to appear as a candidate for the Chair of the Institutions which I had felt in offering myself for that of the Practice of Physic, because I was but too well aware of the efforts which would be made to complete the *arrangement* previously formed for filling up the Medical Chairs which have been lately vacant in the University, and of the nature of the opposition which, as a candidate for a seat in the Medical Faculty, I was likely to encounter, from those with whom this arrangement originated, and to whom its execution appears to have been entrusted; but I was desirous to afford an opportunity to the Patrons of the University of exercising, as independent electors, their right of voting, and to the public of judging of a mode of procedure in the appointment to Chairs in the University, which, while it holds out to candidates the semblance of a fair, candid, and impartial consideration of their testimonials and claims, in reality precludes all honourable competition.[106]

Thomson's response to these disappointments was to withdraw to the extramural school. Together with his elder son William he lectured during the 1820s at his house on George Street on the theory and practice of medicine in direct competition with Home and Alison. He had not, however, abandoned his ambition of gaining a seat in the medical faculty for himself and for his heirs. By 1826 a change in his strategy was evident: having failed to secure one of the existing medical chairs, Thomson took the opportunity of the calling of a Royal Commission on Scottish Universities to argue for the creation of three new professorships.[107]

Hearing that plans for academic reform were under consideration Thomson outlined his ideas on medical education in a pamphlet published under the pseudonym of 'A Graduate of King's College, Aberdeen'. Much of this tract was concerned with the preliminary education that should be required of medical students; but Thomson also raised general questions about the structure of the medical curriculum. He mounted a typically Whig critique of existing arrangements: 'The Schools of Medicine, and the Colleges of Physic and Surgery, which at present exist in Great Britain and Ireland', he complained,

> exhibit many curious anomalies and contradicitions in their Statutes and Practices. Indeed, the examination of the different constitutions of these Corporate Bodies is sufficient to shew that they have not been formed upon any general or enlarged views of public utility, but that monopoly, or privilege of some sort or other, has always been a main object of their establishment.[108]

Traditional institutional forms must, therefore, give way to more rational arrangements especially where the monopoly enjoyed by some individual or group was injurious to the public interest. It was, in particular, Thomson declared

> of great importance to the Public that you should inquire, whether a division of duties among the members of the Medical Faculty, made a century ago, is at all adapted to the conditions of the times in which we live; or calculated to comprehend, and to exhibit to Students, a view, sufficiently complete, of all the discoveries and improvements which have been made in the Theory or in the Practice of Physic, and in those collateral branches of Science, upon the progress of which the advancement of Medicine mainly depends.[109]

Specifically, Thomson asked whether 'the duties at present performed by the Professor of the Theory of Medicine, should not be assigned to two distinct Professors at least – Physiology to one, and Pathology to another?'[110] He was in effect proposing that a new chair of pathology be established while the Professor of the institutes of medicine was restricted to the teaching of physiology. Thomson also raised the old grievance of the need for a separate chair of surgery in the University of Edinburgh.

He repeated this demand in a later pamphlet intended to influence the Royal Commission. He now raised a further issue: the system of clinical instruction in Edinburgh was, Thomson claimed, grossly defective. There was no one professor of clinical medicine; the medical professors instead took it in turn to deliver clinical lectures at the Royal Infirmary. Thomson argued that there was no guarantee that a competent professor of anatomy, chemistry, or botany would also be a good clinical teacher. Moreover, the plurality of professors was likely to confuse the students and to foster the 'unfortunate, because enervating, belief, that Physic is a science in which no fixed principles have yet been, or are likely ever to be, established'.[111] These disadvantages could only be avoided by the foundation of a chair of clinical medicine.

Thomson was well aware that this proposal would meet the same resistance as past efforts to expand the professoriate.[112] But he argued that academic like all other institutions must adapt to meet new conditions. The present arrangements might have been appropriate to an earlier historical epoch; the

> present flourishing condition of this School, however, seems to admit, and the great extension of the boundaries of Medicine seem to require, a further division of labour among the Medical Professors, in order that all the necessary branches of medical knowledge may be taught as fully as possible, and that each Professor may keep pace with the progress of his own department of the Science, and be able to do justice to the numerous pupils committed to his charge.[113]

Thomson's critique of the old academic regime therefore took the form of a rationalist attack upon tradition. In particular, he applied criteria of public utility drawn from the language of political economy to university organization. He thereby stigmatized the present distribution of duties by designating it an example of 'monopoly', while identifying his own calls for a multiplication of chairs with the beneficent and progressive historical process of the division of labour. He also made uncharacteristic use of irony to point out the absurdities of the professoriate's stock response to all plans for innovation. He suggested that in the case of the new chair of music, at least,

> it will not be insisted on, as in the case of other new Professorships, that the duties of that office are already amply fulfilled. The Patrons will not upon this, as upon other similar occasions, be assured by the Senatus Academicus, that the power of Music over the Mind occupies

> no fewer than 8 Lectures in the Course of the Professor of Moral Philosophy, – that its connection with Poetry and Oratory is amply illustrated by the Professor of Rhetoric and Belles Lettres, – that its influence over diseases is insisted on at great length by the Professor of the Practice of Physic, – that the principles of the construction of Musical Instruments are luminously explained by the Professor of Natural Philosophy. – that, by the aid of Hydrogen Gas, and of Tubes of Glass, Earthen-Ware, or Metal the Professor of Chemistry annually produces 'sounds of sweetest melody,' to the infinite delight of the popular part of his audience; and that the Music of the Spheres forms a department of the Course of the Professor of Astronomy, of which he cannot be deprived, without great injustice to himself, and manifest injury to his pupils. On one occasion, at least, we may hope to see each of the Professors cheerfully resigning a portion of his Patrimonial Interests and Vested Rights to promote the Weal and Harmony of the Community.[114]

Thomson rehearsed these arguments in the evidence he gave to the Royal Commission in January 1827.[115] He recognized this as a moment of real opportunity to effect fundamental change in the constitution of the university and exerted himself to seize it. Although he framed these proposals in terms of the public good, it was easy for Thomson's enemies to portray his efforts as motivated by self-interest. As late as 1848 a group of professors alleged that some of the evidence presented to the Commissioners 'was very much designed to favour the views of one gentleman, whose ambition it was at that time to enter the Medical Faculty as Professor of Clinical Medicine'.[116] Thomson had sought to pre-empt such insinuations at the conclusion of his 1826 pamphlet: 'The time has been', he admitted,

> when it might have been supposed that I had a personal interest in recommending the adoption of these measures; but the ambition I long felt of obtaining a seat in the Medical Faculty I now resign to one who has been for some years the associate of my studies, and has been my Assistant in teaching the Practice of Physic.[117]

He thus claimed to have abandoned plans for his own advancement for the hope that William Thomson might achieve a place in the Faculty of Medicine.

Such public disclaimers may provoke scepticism. There is, however, other evidence that by 1827 Thomson was weary and looking to retirement from teaching. He wrote to John Allen that 'If there are to be any new medical chairs established in Glasgow I wish I could get one of them for William. I doubt if I shall lecture another Winter in Edinburgh for the fatigue of it is more than I am able for with the business that presses upon me.' Thomson's mood of depression was reflected also in his remarks upon politics: he beseeched Allen to 'give me what hope you can that the Whigs are to be in power once more before I might quit this scene'.[118] The unexpected fulfilment of this hope was, however, to transform his prospects, and enabled Thomson finally to realize his long-cherished academic ambitions.

General pathology

In December 1830 a Whig government came into office. This event dispelled Thomson's despondency and revived his prospects of preferment. Circumstances were now yet more favourable to him than in 1806; the Edinburgh Whigs with whom he had fraternized at the turn of the century were now among the leaders of the Whig party. In Scotland, Francis Jeffrey was appointed Lord Advocate while Henry Cockburn became Solicitor-General. Moreover, from his base at Holland House, John Allen was singularly well placed to assist his old friend.[119] Even before the final triumph of the Whigs Allen had been able to exercise some influence over academic appointments. In 1827 the Home Secretary Lord Lansdowne (Henry Petty as was) asked for Allen's opinion of the candidates for the vacant chair of botany at Glasgow.[120]

During the spring of 1831 Thomson began to make use of this influence for his own ends. He wrote to Allen to propose the creation of a new chair of general pathology for himself at Edinburgh; at the same time he recruited the help of Macvey Napier, one of the few Whig professors in the university.[121] While Napier undertook to bring the matter to the attention of the Lord Advocate, Allen touted the proposal in London. The decision on such an appointment lay with the Home Secretary, Lord Melbourne, who had as a student in Glasgow lodged with John Millar, and who was sympathetic to Thomson's proposal.

In May, Napier discovered that 'the thing [is] likely to be arranged'; but he also learned that 'nothing had been said as to granting the Commission in such terms as would make Dr Thomson a member of the *Medical Faculty* – a point of the greatest consequence to him'. Thomson had forwarded a draft commission to Allen which did satisfy this requirement; Napier urged Allen to place this document before Melbourne without delay.[122]

From the outset, therefore, Thomson was determined not only to obtain a new chair, but also to ensure that this post would carry with it all the privileges he had so long coveted. Napier realized that a crown commission couched in these terms would represent a break with precedent, and might cause legal problems; a consultation with the Lord Advocate, however, provided some reassurance that these difficulties were not insuperable. In September 1831 Jeffrey advised the Home Office that:

> I have fully considered the application of Dr John Thomson to be appointed Professor of Medicine and General Pathology in the University of Edinburgh – and am humbly of opinion both that the Establishment of such a Professorship would tend to the improvement of the Medical School of that city – and that no person could be found more eminently qualified to fill that station than Dr Thomson.[123]

Jeffrey himself revised the text of Thomson's commission. The new chair was named 'The professorship of Medicine and general Pathology'; the incumbent was thus entitled to give clinical lectures. The commission further stipulated that Thomson was empowered 'to examine Candidates and do every thing that may be required and necessary to the graduation of Doctors of Medicine'.[124] His course was also to be compulsory for those wishing to graduate, a stipulation which was to be the cause of much controversy.

A commission couched in similar terms was at the same time issued to John William Turner making him the first professor of surgery in the University of Edinburgh. Thomson's third proposed innovation – the chair of clinical medicine – was, however, forgotten, perhaps because the terms of his commission as Professor of General Pathology made it redundant.

On hearing of these new appointments, the Senatus Academicus appointed a committee to draw up a response. Only Macvey Napier dissented from this decision.[125] The report presented on 4 October 1831 confined itself to a consideration of Thomson's chair; the committee were of opinion that 'The present appointment of a Professorship of pathology [is] unprecedented in the history of the medical chairs of the University'. They pointed out that the Royal Commission of 1826–7 had not included such an institution in its recommendations. There was, moreover, no pedagogic justification for the measure; pathology was already adequately taught by the existing medical professors. The fact that Thomson was entitled to examine candidates for the MD gave special offence: this was 'a power never before conferred on any Medical Professor by a Commission from the crown'. What made this provision especially alarming was that it might imply that Thomson's course was now part of the requirements for the medical degree.[126] The committee also pointed out that his commission, unlike that of previous Regius professors, contained no clauses preventing 'interference' with the rights of existing professors.[127]

The Town Council was also unhappy. In particular, the right to examine candidates conferred upon Thomson and Turner was seen as an infringement of the control over the university curriculum that the Council had, after lengthy litigation, recently secured. The Council did indicate, however, that these objections might be obviated if the patronage of the new chairs was transferred to them; they therefore petitioned the crown

> that the Commissions granted to these distinguished individuals may be recalled, upon the assurance . . . that they will immediately, as Patrons, issue new Commissions, placing these Professors in the same situation, and under similar regulations as the other members of the Medical Faculty, by adding their classes to the curriculum of study[.][128]

The College Committee of the Council forwarded the report of the Senatus Academicus to Thomson for comment. He took the opportunity to vent some of the resentment he had accumulated over many years of conflict with the professoriate. He alleged that the Senatus had engaged in its late legal action against the Town Council solely

> to shew that there is something so sacred in the character of the Medical Faculty that no foot must enter that sanctuary unless by their express authority and permission; something so delicate in the construction of the Medical Curriculum, that no ruder hands than their own must attempt to repair or improve it.[129]

He quoted Dugald Stewart to show that university professors were, in fact, constitutionally averse to any innovation, adding that

> I have had too frequent occasion in the course of a life, a considerable portion of which has been devoted to the business of teaching Medicine, to notice the unfortunate tendency in our Academical Institutions to remain stationary . . . to feel any great degree of disappointment or mortification at a resistance being made to my humble endeavours to promote the improvement of Medical education at this University.[130]

Given the support from government that he now enjoyed, Thomson could afford to be defiant. When the communications of Town Council and Senatus arrived at the Home Office they were referred to Jeffrey for an opinion. He drew a sharp distinction between the two documents: 'the Memorial of the Magistrates and Council . . . appear to me to be drawn up in a very proper tone and spirit, and so as to make it easy and fitting for the Crown to meet the application by any acts of grace and bounty that may be thought adviseable'. The memorial from the Senatus, on the other hand, was not 'entitled by any means to the same respect and attention'. Jeffrey categorically rejected the university's proposal that the commissions of the new professors be revoked; but he saw no objection to the Town Council's request to be made the patron of the chairs.[131]

The Home Secretary adopted Jeffrey's advice and informed the Lord Provost accordingly.[132] In November 1833 the Council received a royal warrant empowering them to make future appointments to the chairs of surgery and pathology.[133] While this transfer of the patronage of the general pathology chair to the Town Council seemed unexceptionable even to Thomson's friends, it was to prove the cause of much future strife.

Soon after his appointment Thomson began to associate his son William in the teaching of the professorship. Between 1831 and 1836 he also employed James Young Simpson as an assistant.[134] These helpers allowed Thomson to reconcile the requirements of the chair with the demands of private practice. Thus in December 1832 he notified the Lord Provost that

> I have just received an urgent request to visit a old friend of mine in Argyllshire, who is affected with a dangerous disease. As I must necessarily be absent from Edinburgh for five or six days, I have desired my eldest son, Dr W. Thomson, to read my lectures for me till my return, in order that the Students of my class may not sustain any loss by my absence[.][135]

Using his son as a substitute lecturer also served another purpose: this was a time-honoured device by which Scottish professors tried to make their chair hereditary. By October 1836 it was obvious that Thomson was preparing the ground for such a transition.[136] He informed the Town Council that

> the condition of my health still continues to be such as gives me no expectation of being able to teach the class of Pathology during the ensuing Winter Session. In these circumstances, I shall feel it to be necessary to have recourse to the services of my son Dr William Thomson, who is well acquainted with all my opinions relative to Pathology, and in possession of all my manuscripts and illustrative drawings; and who, by his general Medical education, Pathological pursuits, and habits of teaching, I have the satisfaction to believe, is properly qualified for conducting my class.[137]

On 4 July 1837 Thomson finally submitted his resignation. Simpson had no doubt that Thomson planned for his son to succeed him; if the council decided merely to appoint an interim lecturer, he wrote, 'Dr T. says that he shall recommend me to the Council, and not allow William to take it, as it would, in fact, be setting aside his hopes of ever being elected Professor[.]'[138] All these designs were, however, thwarted by an unforeseen turn of events: instead of considering a replacement for Thomson, a faction on the Town Council seconded by the medical faculty argued strenuously for the abolition of the chair of general pathology.

After protracted discussion, the Council on 15 August 1837 forwarded a memorial to the Home Secretary outlining their case for terminating the professorship. They recalled the controversial circumstances under which the chair was founded and argued that the fact that the pathology course was obligatory upon students was particularly objectionable. It increased the burden upon those taking the Edinburgh MD while making the equivalent qualification from Glasgow University correspondingly more attractive: students at Glasgow were only required to attend eight imperative courses as opposed to the fourteen demanded in Edinburgh. As a result, the Council argued, the number of students graduating in Edinburgh had declined by 26 per cent since the institution of the general pathology class. During the same period graduations in Glasgow had risen by nearly 200 per cent.[139] Given the economic importance of the university to the city,

> whatever is injurious to the one is necessarily injurious to the other, and . . . whatever has a tendency to promote the prosperity of the one promotes the prosperity of the other. As guardians of the interests of the City, as well as in their character of patron of the University, your Memorialists therefore respectfully urge Her Majesty's Government to acquiesce in the abolition of the Chair of General Pathology as a separate class.[140]

Four members of the medical faculty had, with the approval of their colleagues, supported this appeal by undertaking to teach a course of general pathology themselves so eliminating the need for a separate professor. The proceeds of this course would go towards a pension for Thomson.[141]

The Thomsons saw John Allen as their best defence against this onslaught. William Thomson complained to him that

> the Town Council look on University degrees as a portion of the *Common Good* of the City, out of which as much profit as possible must be made; and that the terms of granting these degrees must be regulated by the prices of competing traders.

The relatively greater popularity of Glasgow to Edinburgh had, he maintained, nothing to do with the establishment of the chair of general pathology:

> I am sorry to say that so far as I can learn there prevails at Glasgow an exceedingly lax system of Examination; so that it is believed that men rejected here, repair to Glasgow, and find no difficulty in getting through there.

There was therefore much room for improvement in Glasgow; but this was no reason 'to deteriorate the Edinburgh education with a view to bring the two Universities upon a nearer footing of equality'. Thomson was scathing also about the attitude of the Edinburgh professoriate. The students, he claimed, who had attended general pathology were well satisfied with the course: 'I know, however, that great pains have been taken by several of the Professors, both at their private houses and in the Wards of the Infirmary, to poison the minds of the Students on the matter'.[142]

Allen forwarded Thomson's letter to the Home Secretary, Lord John Russell. As well as urging Russell to resist demands for the abolition of the general pathology chair, Allen sought to broaden the discussion to a general consideration of the state of the Scottish universities; the immediate issue merely illustrated the urgent necessity of reform.[143] In a similar vein Allen told Macvey Napier that 'The proceedings of the Town Council in the affair of the Pathological Chair shew the incompetence of a body so constituted and appointed to regulate schools for science .... The University must perish in such hands.'[144]

Allen confessed himself baffled by the hostility to Thomson in Edinburgh. From his position in London he was oblivious to the degree of resentment that the original institution of the general pathology chair had generated. In Edinburgh the creation of the chair was seen as a peculiarly gross example of political favouritism: one councillor declared that 'It was almost universally believed that the creation of this Chair, in 1831, was a job.'[145] Robert Knox in an open letter to the Lord Provost was still more outspoken. The establishment of the surgery and pathology chairs was, in his view, 'a political job of the very worst description'. As an extramural lecturer, Knox also objected to the monopolistic powers given to the new professors.[146] In a later letter he referred to the 'notorious and odious manner in which the Chairs of General Pathology and Surgery were originally instituted'.[147] An anonymous pamphleteer epitomized these sentiments about the foundation of the pathology chair when he declared that 'if [Thomson] had not been a favourite with some of the famed intriguers at Holland House, his peculiar merits as a teacher would have remained either undiscovered or neglected'.[148]

Despite this local hostility, the issue of the survival of the pathology chair was finally decided by the ministry in London. Lord John Russell was an old associate of Edinburgh Whigs and a good friend to the Thomson family. In his response to the Town Council's memorial, Russell adopted many of William Thomson's arguments; he insisted that

> if the Government wish to advance the interests of Science and secure to the Public the advantages of high Professional knowledge their course should be not to lower the course of study in Edinbro' to the level of Glasgow or any other of the Scotch Universities but to endeavour to raise them to the higher standard.

Were the Town Council's contentions valid, 'the cheapest education [should be] considered as synonimous with the best'.[149] Russell accordingly refused either to countenance the abolition of the pathology chair or to render it unnecessary to graduation.

John Thomson had repaired to London in order to lobby ministers. From there he wrote to the Lord Provost on 29 September withdrawing his resignation. He was to remain in his chair until 1842 when ill-health finally forced his retirement. Although the general pathology chair was safe, Thomson ultimately failed to see it pass to his son. Thomson's growing infirmity obliged him to rely on William to teach his course. He expressed the hope that 'my Son's lecturing for me, under these circumstances, will not prove a bar to his being recognised as a Candidate for the Chair of Pathology when it shall become vacant'.[150] This was a forlorn hope. Thomson was advised that

> the Council do not acquiesce in his wish that any Gentleman who has been or may be appointed an Interim Lecturer to conduct the Class of Pathology, after the declaration on the part of Dr Thomson, that he did not expect ever to be able to resume teaching the Class, shall be eligible to become a Candidate for that Chair in the event of a Vacancy.[151]

The Town Council had at least ensured that the obnoxious pathology chair would not remain the property of the Thomson family.

Conclusion

It may appear anomalous that in the midst of teaching, practice and politics, John Thomson should have found the time to begin and partially complete his life of Cullen. This enterprise was, however, no mere act of disinterested scholarship, but was continuous with and supportive of Thomson's other endeavours. The biography of a famous medical professor physician served, in the first place, to reinforce the professional persona Thomson sought to develop during the 1820s. Work on the biography provided him with materials to deploy in his polemics: for instance Cullen's views were cited as authority for a proposed division of the responsibilities of the chair of the institutes of medicine.[152] The *Life* also gave Thomson an opportunity to present his views on such matters as medical education to a wide readership and to claim Cullen's concurrence in some of his opinions.[153]

Thomson's account of Cullen's career, moreover, sometimes contains elements of autobiography. His remarks on Cullen as a clinical teacher cast light, for example, on why Thomson was so eager to secure the right to give clinical lectures at the Edinburgh military hospitals:

> Besides possessing high qualifications as a clinical lecturer, Dr Cullen had the strongest motives to employ all the powers of his mind in this new field of professional exertion. His lectures on clinical medicine afforded the most favourable opportunity that could be desired of exhibiting publicly in Edinburgh his talents as a teacher of medicine, of evincing his skill and experience as a practical physician, and of establishing by those means a claim to the chair of the practice of physic, when it should become vacant[.][154]

But it is in the remarks on the opposition Cullen met in Edinburgh that these autobiographical references are most obvious. On one occasion, Thomson reported, 'Cullen was so much disgusted with the conduct of the Patrons of the University, and with the treatment he had received, that, on the death of Dr Whytt, he seems to have wished to remain Professor of Chemistry'.[155] When recounting Cullen's eventual accession to the practice chair, Thomson did not neglect to underline the point:

> Such were the difficulties to be overcome, and such the exertions required to procure, first, a place in the University of Edinburgh, and afterwards the proper situation in it, for the man whose genius, talents and industry shed such lustre over the Institution, and contributed in so remarkable a degree to extend and to perpetuate the fame of its Medical School![156]

This chapter has recounted the difficulties that Thomson had to overcome and the exertions required to obtain a place for himself in the Faculty of Medicine of Edinburgh University. Unlike Cullen, he achieved this only by using his political influence to create a new chair for himself. Thomson was drawing to the end of his active professional life by the time he attained this goal and was unable fully to enjoy it: he never exercised the privilege of acting as a clinical professor although he did serve as an examiner. Perhaps most galling was that Thomson failed to bequeath his seat in the Faculty to his son.

After a further period of extramural teaching in Edinburgh, William Thomson was obliged to be content with a chair in Glasgow. The indispensable John Allen (to whom the *Life of Cullen* was dedicated) again played his part, giving assurance that William Thomson was 'well qualified for the Chair and will make a good Teacher, and that in politicks he is all [the Glasgow MPs] could desire'. He was 'a good Whig and was so when Whigs had little chance of being ever in a situation to have professorships to bestow'.[157]

John Thomson did, however, live to see a kind of eventual triumph. In 1842 his younger son Allen was appointed professor of the institutes of medicine at Edinburgh – one of the chairs to which Thomson had himself unsuccessfully aspired. His ambition to see a Thomson in one of the ancient medical chairs of the university was thus fulfilled.

4

Pathologists and practitioners

Introduction

John Thomson was an example of a particular kind of medical practitioner in nineteenth-century Britain. These men sought to combine the role of teacher with that of clinician. Their clinical activities can be further analysed into attendance upon public hospitals and the treatment of private patients. In Edinburgh with its large medical school the possibilities of a career as an academic clinician were especially obvious. A community of such practitioners can be identified in the city in the first half of the nineteenth century; the relative weight given to the different elements of this compound role differed, however, between individuals.

Complex reciprocal relationships existed between teaching and practice. Teaching could provide a young doctor with a useful source of income while he sought to build up a practice. John Allen's course on the animal oeconomy, for instance, was in part intended to perform this function (see chapter 2). In that case, however, the anticipated patients never appeared; the course itself failed to attract auditors in sufficient numbers to provide Allen with a living; and he was eventually obliged to leave Edinburgh.

Teaching could also serve as a form of advertising for a rising practitioner. It brought him before the eye of the public as an accomplished member of the profession to whom patients might with confidence bring their afflictions. A reputation as a successful lecturer might thus make a man a fashionable practitioner. Chairs in the medical faculty of the university – and especially those that carried the right to give clinical lectures – were especially valuable in establishing such a reputation.

This strategy for professional success presupposed that potential patients as well as students would be impressed and attracted by a particular persona. The academic clinician presented himself as one with a philosophical understanding of medicine: as someone who delved into the principles and causes that underlay the phenomena of health and disease. To establish this identity fully it was necessary to do more than merely retail facts and theories derived from others; the true philosophic practitioner himself contributed to the growth of medical knowledge. Andrew Duncan signalled his awareness of this desideratum at the outset of his lectures on the institutes of medicine when he declared that, as well as recounting received facts, 'I shall endeavour to establish a new Doctrine, *the Universality of a Coagulable Matter, thro' the whole Animal System*.'[1] The importance attached to such alleged innovations was evident in the fiercely proprietorial attitudes displayed by those who maintained that they had made new contributions. Perhaps the best known example is the acrimonious priority dispute between Alexander Monro II and the Hunters over the discovery of the absorbent system.

By making such claims to have advanced science, the teacher sought admission to an international community of savants who perused and appraised each other's work. He addressed this audience through his publications. As well as students and patients the philosophical practitioner thus also looked for the approval of his peers in the world of medical science.

The demands of these diverse groups of patrons did not necessarily conflict; but it could prove difficult simultaneously to satisfy them all. Individual practitioners decided how to reconcile these different calls upon their time and attention. In the course of a lifetime, this system of priorities could be revised. The conventional view was that teaching was most important early in a man's career. As his practice grew, so he had less time to devote to lecturing and less need of student fees. Not all subscribed, however, to this purely instrumental and mercenary view of the place of pedagogy in a medical career; Charles Bell asserted that 'I have always maintained that the most useful and honorable condition of a medical man was when he joined teaching with consultation – in preference to the whirl and incessant motion of a London physician – tied to his Chariot wheels.'[2]

John Thomson's career conformed closely to the main lineaments of this general type. From around 1800 he pursued teaching and practice in parallel. As the character of one of these activities changed the other was modified accordingly. He also undertook original researches and encouraged others to do likewise. The publication of the results of some of these enquiries in 1813 secured Thomson a European reputation as a medical savant.[3] He was recognized by eminent continental researchers like Friedrich Tiedemann;[4] and, conversely, he revealed a familiarity with French and German as well as British contributions to medical science.

It is, however, impossible to establish any clear hierarchy among the pursuits that constituted Thomson's professional identity. On two occasions early in his career he abandoned private practice to enable him 'to be able to devote my time exclusively to the learning and teaching of Surgery'.[5] Such ostensible devotion to the cause of medical education at the expense of personal gain could serve to establish a character as a public-spirited citizen which might redound to Thomson's advantage.

Writing of Thomson's efforts as professor of surgery at the RCS, Patrick Erskine in 1806 maintained that it was

> no slight consideration, that, in order to do justice to this very important course, he has withdrawn himself, for a time at least, from private family practice; on which account, he may be considered as fairly entitled to every support and encouragement that can with propriety be offered him; and, in that view, the institution of the Professorship [of military surgery] would not only be a measure of great general utility, but . . . would also be an act of justice to a most useful servant of the Public.[6]

Thomson did eventually return to private practice with considerable success. But he did not abandon teaching even when it became difficult to reconcile the demands of lecturing with the requirements of patients. Instead Thomson sought to raise his son William to be a surrogate lecturer who would relieve him of some of the load. To the end of his career, however, pedagogy remained central to Thomson's professional identity.

Thomson's scientific activity also possessed close connections with the other strands of his career. The new doctrines that he developed were displayed in the first instance to his students. He also encouraged them to pursue similar investigations in the context of the Royal Medical Society, for the probationary essays they were required to write for the fellowship of the RCS, or for their MD disseratations.[7] The publication of Thomson's researches could also, by strengthening his claims to be an erudite and profound medical thinker, further his ambitions as a clinician: when acknowledging receipt of Thomson's *Lectures on Inflammation* Matthew Baillie remarked that 'I should think that it must lead to that kind of practice which would be most agreeable to you, viz. the business of consultation.'[8]

None of the three aspects of Thomson's professional activity was dominant over the others. Instead a synergy existed between them: each contributing to and receiving some reinforcement from the rest. The interplay of these flows constituted Thomson as a medical man. They also shaped the fortunes of those who came within his field of influence. The remainder of this chapter will consider these relations in more detail.

The rational and scientific surgeon

From the outset John Thomson's attempts to establish himself as teacher and practitioner in Edinburgh were enmeshed in controversy and conflict. He obtained the post of surgeon-in-ordinary at the Royal Infirmary in 1800 after a bitter dispute over the proper way of organizing surgical attendance at the hospital.[9] The furore caused by his appointment in 1804 as professor of surgery at the RCS has been described above.

This controversial debut was to have long-term consequences for Thomson both as a surgeon and as a teacher of surgery. In 1808–9 his competence as a surgeon was challenged by John Bell; as a result of these allegations, Thomson was obliged to resign from his position at the Royal Infirmary.[10] Bell had been the chief antagonist of Thomson's party in the dispute over surgical attendance.

The contentious circumstances in which Thomson's chair at the Royal College of Surgeons was created also carried a legacy. They imposed a number of polemical imperatives upon him which structured the content of his teaching. It was first incumbent upon him to demonstrate that his role was not superfluous: to refute the claim that the need for surgical instruction in Edinburgh was already adequately supplied by the professor of anatomy. In short, Thomson was obliged to show that he had a distinctive and vital contribution to make to medical education in the city.

He based his argument upon the fact that the Monros lectured only on the operations of surgery. This in Thomson's view reflected a misconception that surgery consisted essentially in a set of manual skills – that it was a 'mere handycraft'. He argued that, on the contrary,

> Surgery is not as has been represented merely the art of curing diseases by external remedies and by manual operation, nor must we imagine as but too many people have done that when a man has learned the art of dressing Sores, of applying Bandages and performing operations with a little dexterity that he must be an accomplished Surgeon – He who would practice Surgery with probity and success must study it both as a science and as an art, for a man destitute of principles is little better than a Surgical automaton, while the man of mere Erudition can only be considered as a learned Spectator.[11]

In place of the artisan-surgeon, Thomson sought to erect the ideal of the *scientific* surgeon.

The notion of scientific surgery was not Thomson's invention. Ironically it owed much to the writings of one of his enemies. John Bell, in the course of his controversy with James Gregory, argued that surgery was a 'demonstrative science' not an empirical art. Surgery possessed this status because its rational practice was based upon an intimate knowledge of the structure of the body in health and disease. Experience of dissection gave the trainee operator a certain manual dexterity; this, however, was the least of anatomy's uses to the surgeon. Anatomy was also 'the grounds of all argument, on questions of practice; it connects the senses, with the reason'. In particular, the surgeon's knowledge of the changes produced in the organs by disease 'enables him to prescribe, to consult, and to decide, on the more difficult questions submitted to his judgment'.[12]

In his lectures Thomson gave due emphasis to surgical anatomy. He expatiated, for example, upon the relations between the skull, dura mater, and brain; a knowledge of these structures was held to be important in performing the operation for the trepan.[13] He also demonstrated surgical operations on cadavers to the students. But for Thomson mere anatomy was too narrow an intellectual basis for surgery. While Bell concentrated his remarks upon operative surgery, Thomson employed a much more commodious conception of surgical practice. 'In Surgery', he wrote,

> we only have recourse to an operation when there is great danger & urgency. Operations are dangerous & painful but we must also attend to the previous & subsequent treatment[.] The knowledge of Anatomy is absolutely necessary. But the most difficult part is to know where an operation should be performed & when a disease can be cured without an operation[.][14]

In short, surgeons were more concerned with the medical treatment of surgical diseases than with the performance of operations; they were 'not to estimate our knowledge from the number of operations we have performed, or the number of our fellow creatures we have mutilated but rather from the number of lives we have saved without having recourse to operation'.[15]

The rational foundation of this, the more important part of surgical practice, lay not in anatomy, but in a sound knowledge of pathology. Thomson highlighted this pathological dimension to his teaching from the outset of his career: in the prospectus to the course of lectures on military surgery that he delivered in the spring of 1804 he announced that 'the Attention of the Student will be particularly directed to the Pathology of the different injuries, and to the Reasons for which Operations or Medicines, recommended in the Treatment of them, are to be employed'.[16] Thomson was consistent in this emphasis; he taught pathology in Edinburgh long before the subject achieved any official status in the medical curriculum.

This distinctive conception of the scope of surgical pedagogy helped to vindicate Thomson's appointment: he could claim that his teaching satisfied needs ignored by other lecturers. It also served wider polemical purposes. On several occasions in his lectures Thomson referred to the Royal College of Surgeons as 'my patrons'. His course was mounted in their premises and under their protection; in return he sought to serve the interests of the College. Thomson's concept of scientific surgery was fully consistent with the learned and genteel image that the Edinburgh surgeons had since the 1770s attempted to project.

The extended concept of surgery he promulgated had the further advantage of corresponding with the realities of practice confronting his students.

Most would go on to be general practitioners, not 'pure' surgeons. Those destined for military or naval service would, in particular, be expected to minister to all the medical needs of large populations of patients. Even in such an *echt* surgical matter as the treatment of wounds, febrile symptoms might supervene; the surgeon needed therefore to be familiar with the nature and treatment of constitutional as well as local disease.

The very distinction between surgery and physic was threatened. In Thomson's scheme 'surgery' encompassed virtually the whole of medical practice. He took pains to draw out these implications. He gave his students a lengthy historical account of the development of medical institutions in Europe since ancient times to show that the division between surgery and physic was wholly arbitrary.[17] On the other hand, the basic *unity* of the healing art on which he insisted had its basis in the nature of disease itself: constitutional and local affections were inextricably linked. As late as 1832 Thomson continued to insist upon this point. In the *Life of Cullen* he wrote that

> When separate colleges of physicians and surgeons began to be established in the different countries of Europe, attempts were made to ascertain and to establish by law the particular limits of these two professions. In making these attempts, however, Governments had undertaken a task far beyond their powers, the object of them being quite irreconcilable with the laws which nature observes in the production, course, complications, and cure, of local and constitutional diseases.[18]

By eliding the distinction between physic and surgery Thomson was able to repudiate the notion that the physician was inherently superior to the surgeon. Indeed, at times he seemed to suggest that the conventional hierarchy should be inverted: if, he argued,

> this view of the proper objects of Physic and Surgery, and of the means which the physician and Surgeon respectively employ in the cure of diseases be just, it is obvious that Surgery must form by far the most extensive and important branch of the healing art. For a knowledge of this branch implies you perceive not only an acquaintance with local diseases and manual operations, but also with the phenomena, pathology and treatment of those constitutional affections to which local diseases give rise and by which they are so frequently accompanied in their progress.

In view of the importance of surgery to the art and science of medicine it was 'strange . . . that in the Academical arrangements which have been formed in this Country to facilitate the study of Medicine no particular provision should have been made for teaching Surgery'. It was to remedy this defect that 'My Patrons the Royal College and Incorporation of Surgeons' had instituted Thomson's chair.[19]

There are parallels between the polemical function served by pathology within Thomson's scheme and events in contemporary France. There the doctrine that there was 'only one pathology' legitimated the recent, and still controversial, unification of the medical profession that had occurred in the aftermath of the Revolution. Pathology was presented as a single body of knowledge underpinning both physic and surgery.[20] Although no formal amalgamation had occurred in Edinburgh, Thomson argued that there was a *de facto* unity dependent upon a set of shared concepts and practices.

It was one thing to assert that 'pathology' was the basis of all rational medical practice and quite another to supply some account of the content of that science. The term was in a state of flux in the early decades of the nineteenth century with venerable competing with more recent significations. Thomson was aware of this indeterminancy of meaning: in his lectures he distinguished a number of different conceptions of pathology that had existed in the past, some of which still persisted. Prominent among these were systems that ascribed all ailments to some single proximate cause; as examples, Thomson listed the doctrines of Cullen and John Brown, adding at a later date the theories of François-Joseph-Victor Broussais to the list. He was dismissive of pathology of this variety: 'In constructing these Pathological Theories', he maintained, 'much labour has been thrown away in investigating subjects placed by nature beyond the reach of the Human Faculties.'[21]

Sound theories of disease could only be based upon a knowledge of phenomena accessible to the senses – not upon such hypothetical causes as 'Lentor, and viscidity, . . . obstruction, . . . Acrimony, . . . Plethora, and Spasm, . . . [and] vigour and Debility'. In this regard surgeons were much more reliable pathologists than were physicians. Surgery had 'kept free from that unmeaning jargon which Medical pathologists have but too often used in the explanation of morbid phenomena'. There was, Thomson argued, a special surgical mentality which militated against such fallacies:

> The phenomena and change of structure which occur in Surgical diseases, being obvious to the senses, the Surgical pathologist is necessarily limited in his discription [*sic*] of these changes to sensible objects, to objects too definite and precise to leave any room for the exercise of the imagination, and too plain to receive any illustration from the adoption of vague, inconsistent and erroneous hypothetical explanations.[22]

The most salient feature of the distinctively surgical approach to the understanding of disease was the impulse to search for localized lesions with which symptoms could be correlated. This mode of pathological investigation had been 'of late years cultivated with great ardor in this country as well as upon the Continent, and large and most interesting additions have been made to our stock of pathological knowledge'.[23]

Thomson's description of the history and tendency of pathology at the turn of the nineteenth century accords well with later accounts. It confirms both the notion of the rise of pathological anatomy and the claim that the presuppositions underlying this mode of conceptualizing disease had roots in the special characteristics of surgical thought.[24] For Thomson, however, these arguments performed a polemical function: they served to identify surgery with progressive movements in contemporary medicine while belittling the contribution of physicians.

Thomson established for himself a reputation as a surgeon-pathologist at the forefront of contemporary developments in science. He was, in particular, credited with introducing the leading concepts of the new French pathology to British medicine and for accommodating these to the native traditions of the Hunterian school. An examination of Thomson's lecture notes reveals several levels to his pathological discourse. The first of these may be considered as surgical pathology narrowly defined. He gave, for example, a detailed account of the malformations associated with cleft palate with a practical view in mind: although there was nothing to be done for the palate itself, in extreme cases where the lip itself was split the surgeon could effect union. Thomson provided an account of this operation directly after his discussion of the pathology of the condition.

A second strand comprised classical organ pathology as expounded by Morgagni or Matthew Baillie. From an early date, however, Thomson showed an awareness of the major revolution in conceptualizing the seats of disease that had recently occurred. He emphasized to his students that

> not only is the Human body composed of numerous organs, but every individual organ in the animal economy is itself composed of several textures, which differ widely from each other in their vital Physical and Chemical properties. Such undoubtedly are skin, cellular membrane, artery, vein, absorbent, nerve, muscle, tendon, ligament, cartilage, and bone. These textures differing so widely from one another in structure, it is reasonable to believe that they will differ also in the diseases to which they are liable.[25]

Thomson thus adopted the system of general anatomy propounded by 'the late most ingenious Professor Bichat of Paris'. The task of pathological anatomy was to describe the morbid changes that occurred at the level of the constituent tissues of the body. It was this investigation, which had already been pursued with much success in France, that 'promises to banish from the Schools of Medicine those fanciful and futile Hypotheses with regard to the nature and cure of diseases with which they have been so long, and so unprofitably occupied'.[26]

An insistence upon the localization of disease in the component tissues of the body was recognized by contemporaries as a distinctive feature of Thomson's thought.[27] In his lectures he paid special attention to the affections of the several component structures of the skin – a subject neglected by other Edinburgh teachers. In 1819 he delivered a separate course on diseases of the eye and even contemplated specializing in the treatment of these complaints.[28]

Thomson took care, however, to describe the limits of localism. Certain morbid processes were universal to all parts of the body although they might undergo modifications in specific textures. Other complaints were purely functional and left no lesion.[29] Moreover, even when particular tissues were affected, it was necessary for the pathologist to take a more comprehensive view of the effects of disease. The different parts of which the human body was composed were, Thomson declared,

> arranged so as to form an entire whole system the parts of which act, and are reciprocally acted on by each other, and tho' some morbid alterations of Structure may disturb the general Constitution so little as to be attended with Symptoms too slight for observation, yet there are other local diseases which often produce Constitutional effects of the most alarming and fatal nature.

It was 'in the knowledge and treatment of these and similar diseases that the boundaries which divide Surgery from Physic meet, and are lost in one another'.[30]

Pathology therefore transcended pathological anatomy just as surgery transcended the treatment of topical disease. The constitutional effects of disease had to be studied by other means. Here the expertise in chemistry that Thomson had gained in his early years in Edinburgh was of service. In his discussion of ailments of the urinary tract, for instance, he did not confine himself to the morbid alterations found at autopsy; he discussed the chemical changes associated with these diseases. Thus he gave his students an account of the normal composition of urine, and then described how this was modified in such diseases as diabetes. In the process he gave a glimpse of how he combined pathological investigation with his clinical work: 'I once evaporated several pounds of the Urine of a Patient labouring under this disease who made on average 10 and 12 and obtained little else besides a few Crystals of the Muriate of Soda.'[31] Thomson had also attended to the morbid anatomy of the condition but found it of limited use to the pathologist:

> Little apparent change is produced upon the Kidnies by this disease. From my own observations and the concurrent Testimony of Several

> Authors who have made accurate Dissections I believe I may affirm that the Structure of the Kidneys of diabetic patients is softer, more vascular and the Tubuli Uriniferi more dilated than in healthy Kidnies.[32]

In the course of his discussion Thomson touched upon some current issues in physiology which were relevant to an understanding of the disease. 'The great point at present in dispute among Medical men', he remarked, 'is about the organs in which the Sugar is generated.' Pathological enquiries could also give rise to new physiological problems: 'In the course of the investigation respecting Diabetes it has become a question whether the Urine ought to be regarded as a Secretion properly so called or merely as a Separation from the blood of principles formerly existing in it'. Urea at least should, in Thomson's view, be recognized as a true secretion manufactured in the kidney.[33]

The propriety of such an extended discussion of organic chemistry in a course on surgery might be questioned; but Thomson maintained that these topics were of immediate value to the practitioner. After an account of the various salts contained in the urine he remarked, 'The fact that these substances are Soluble in different Menstrua shows how nugatory every attempt must be to discover an Universal Solvent or general internal remedy for the Stone.' On the other hand, the same discovery,

> by making us acquainted with the Chemical qualities of the different Species of Calculi and with the Reagents by which they may be dissolved out of the body has afforded us ground to believe that the nature of the calculus being known we may perhaps retard its growth and in some instances even effectuate its dissolution.[34]

If this hope were to be realized, however, the surgeon needed to possess an intimate knowledge of the chemistry of the subject.

The chemical instruction Thomson provided was, moreover, not merely theoretical; it is clear from his notes that he performed some chemical demonstrations before the students. He was in general ready to employ a variety of techniques to make his teaching attractive to his audience. Thomson shared with other Edinburgh professors an approach to pedagogy in which spectacle of various kinds was used to enhance and enliven lectures.[35]

Thomson was instrumental in creating a pathological museum at the Royal College of Surgeons, and used the preparations it contained to illustrate his lectures.[36] His teaching was, however, more especially distinguished by the extensive use he made in his lectures of coloured delineations of morbid structures. Thomson maintained that these gave a much more vivid representation of disease than any preserved specimen. He first began to employ this technique as a professor of surgery. Thomson initially took advantage of the depictions published by others: diseases of the eye were particularly well covered by such authors as Beer, Demours, Adams and Wardrop.[37] Increasingly, however, these resources seemed inadequate to his needs. Between 1814 and 1819 he employed John Alexander Schetky, a half-pay army surgeon and former student, to produce 'several anatomical and pathological drawings'; the latter illustrated aspects of both internal and external pathology.[38] Later he recruited Robert Carswell to undertake the same task on a much more extensive scale.[39]

In his introductory lecture Thomson tried to show why illustrations were essential to learning pathology. He argued that they provided a direct visual representation of disease which was free of the ambiguities and confusions attendant upon language. Thus, while appreciative of the merits of John Abernethy's treatise on tumours,[40] Thomson expressed the wish that 'his essay had been accompanied with a few drawings similar to those with which Dr Baillie has illustrated his work on Morbid Anatomy'. Such illustrations were no mere diversions from the text but constitutive of a proper understanding of the pathology. Anyone who

> read Mr Abernethy's descriptions and who at the same time [looked] into an account of a tumour described of late years by Mr Burns of Glasgow under the name of Spongoid inflammation and by Mr Hey of Leeds . . . by the name of Fungus Haematodes will I conceive agree with me in thinking that descriptions alone are insufficient to give accurate conceptions of morbid structures, and that drawings plain or coloured are indispensibly necessary to render descriptions of which we have every reason to believe the accuracy even barely intelligible.[41]

In the case of fungus haematodes, this need had, Thomson added, been lately supplied by a work by his friend James Wardrop.[42]

Illustrations therefore stamped order on to the babel of mere words. They made possible that ready and uniform association between name and appearance essential to the formation of a disciplined and scientific profession. Definitive pictures of disease would ensure that all Thomson's students saw the same thing when they uttered a term like 'fungus haematode'. Thomson's epistemology therefore embodied an elevation of the ocular to a position of paramount importance; the pictures he employed in his teaching purported to preserve the truths about disease accessible to the trained pathological eye.[43]

A number of the illustrations Thomson used in his lectures survive and directions scattered in his lecture notes give an indication of how they were employed. Sometimes they served to elucidate normal structures: thus he used one series of plates to illustrate the relations between the membranes of the brain.[44] More usually, the depictions were of manifestations of disease. Several of them were devoted to affections of the skin. Thomson was to 'shew the Girl's face' when discussing inflammation of cellular tissue; and to 'shew figure' illustrating a carbuncle of the back.[45] Others depicted such internal complaints as adhesive inflammation of serous membranes of the lungs. The latter picture in particular was heavily theory-laden: it provided a graphic embodiment of the new tissue pathology.

By 1820 Thomson had begun to think of mounting a course solely on morbid anatomy organized around these illustrations. This would, however, require a vastly larger supply of drawings than he possessed. Carswell was set to work to meet this requirement. But the collection of such a pedagogic resource was dependent upon access to a copious supply of pathological material for the artist to depict; and such an abundance of models was not to be found in Edinburgh. Thomson's great undertaking had to be accomplished elsewhere.

Foreign parts

The exodus to France of British medical students in the aftermath of the Napoleonic Wars to study new clinical and pathological techniques has been documented by Maulitz and others. John Thomson's role in encouraging students from Edinburgh to make this journey has also been recognized.[46] Less well appreciated is the degree to which these missions abroad were an extension of Thomson's domestic designs. Not only Carswell but both Thomson's sons were in the 1820s sent to the Continent for prolonged periods with the express aim of collecting illlustrations and specimens to advance their patron's Edinburgh teaching. They were, in effect, gathering the raw materials from which John Thomson intended to manufacture a science of general pathology in Britain.

It was, above all, the *quantity* of material available to the pathologist that made France such an important resource in this endeavour. When reviewing recent French writings on hernia Thomson remarked that 'The great opportunities which these anatomists have enjoyed of dissecting dead subjects . . . have enabled them to add most valuable contributions to our knowledge of the pathology of this disease.'[47]

Thomson was himself a pioneer channel crosser. In the summer of 1814, he availed himself of the end of hostilities 'to execute a purpose he had long had at heart'. Armed with a letter of introduction from Dugald Stewart and in the company of two medical friends he made his first trip to the continent.[48] According to Robert Renton, one of his companions,

> In the course of this journey, we visited France, Italy, Austria, Saxony, Prussia, Hanover, and Holland, where we examined minutely into the modes of Medical and Surgical Practice followed in the public hospitals of those countries.

Thomson also took full advantage of the opportunities for pathological instruction on offer: Renton was struck by 'The minute accuracy . . . with which he examined the Anatomical and Pathological collections at the Ecole de Medicine in Paris, at Pavia, Vienna, Berlin, Leipsic, Hallé, Gottingen Amsterdam, and Leyden.' Such devotion 'evinced an ardour in his researches, which I and my fellow traveller . . . could not observe but with feelings of surprise and admiration'.[49]

As usual, Thomson's activities abroad were directly linked with his Edinburgh strategy. The clinical and pathological observations he made on the Continent were, he told his wife, to contribute to a textbook on physic and surgery he planned to write upon his return. He also planned to open a '*Clinicum* for the poor. . . . This clinicum will give me the means of observing and of describing the different diseases which I shall occasion to give an account of in my Outlines of Physic and Surgery'.[50] Although Thomson's textbook never appeared, the latter plan came to fruition when Thomson helped to found the New Town Dispensary in Edinburgh.[51]

The journal Thomson kept during his travels confirms Renton's remarks. One afternoon at the Ecole de Médecine he spent 'upwards of two hours in examining their collection of diseased bones'; although there were some fine specimens, Thomson thought the collection to be on the whole inferior to those he had seen in London and Edinburgh.[52] He revealed his interest in the technologies of medical representation when he noted that 'some diseases are here very well imitated in wax, but I do not from what I have seen admire much this form of representing diseases unless for very young students'.[53]

The same day he had visited the Hôpital Saint-Louis, which specialized in the treatment of skin diseases. He conversed with its director, J.L. Alibert, who 'very civilly invited me to look at his plates and drawings'.[54] Thomson was, however, disappointed in his hope of viewing large numbers of patients suffering from chest complaints: he told his wife that 'The beds in the Hospitals destined for these diseases are at present occupied with wounded soldiers.'[55]

Thomson also introduced himself to other prominent Parisian men of science and medicine, including Georges Cuvier,[56] Jean Esquirol, and Philippe Pinel. He took the opportunity of his visit to deepen his acquaintance with their work. Thomson thought the Jardin des Plantes, 'the most splendid thing I have yet seen. I looked over the fossile bones of which Cuvier has given so full a description.'[57] While, after he had visited the Salpêtrière and 'had another interview with the insane', Thomson felt that 'I shall read Pinel's work on Insanity with more pleasure . . . because I am satisfied from what I have seen that I shall understand him better'.[58]

Such professional avocations did not, however, exhaust Thomson's energies. He socialized with other British visitors to the French capital including Lord and Lady Holland with whom he dined 'en famille'.[59] He also found time to go to the opera-house – an experience which left a lasting impression on a man used to a more austere culture:

> the music Dancing and spectacle were much finer than any thing of the kind I had ever seen. It lasted too long for me. The Dancers were all dressed either naked, or so as to appear so, the women having on only a gauze petticoat through which you could see their shapes very well –[60]

Thomson also found amusement and edification in less obvious places. Having obtained a ticket to visit the institute for the blind and deaf from the philosopher Joseph Marie de Gérando,

> I was much gratified by the progress which they have made in learning different trades, Arts and sciences – One of the most interesting parts of the entertainment was a conversation carried on between a deaf and dumb man & one perfectly blind – the deaf & dumb man spoke with his fingers & the blind man with his tongue. A little blind Girl played delightfully on the Piano-forte.[61]

Thomson also took an interest in French politics. A visit to the Corps Legislatif enabled him the opportunity to patronize France's faltering first steps to representative government: the French, he declared, 'are not yet prepared for [debate], nor for many other blessings which our constitution gives'.[62] He later attended a discussion of press freedom and 'lost four hours in listening to the reading of a schoolboy exercise. You need have no expectations from the House of Deputies. They are all poor and place hunters.'[63]

Thomson found less diversion in the other European cities he visited but concentrated on his medical and scientific interests. When in Vienna he showed a special interest in surgery, noting the techniques employed in operations for crural hernia and lithotomy.[64] Berlin was notable for its museums: 'The preparations of natural structure were numerous and beautiful', while the collections of morbid anatomy contained specimens that cast light on several contentious questions in pathology. Thomson also took the opportunity to visit Berlin's Military Hospital.[65] The treatment of syphilis in Prague chiefly attracted Thomson's attention; but he also inspected the 'small but interesting collection of pathological preparations'. The museum contained, he noted, 'several well coloured delineations of disease also'.[66]

In some ways Thomson's 1814 grand tour was the model for the later, much more extensive and protracted expeditions undertaken by his protégés. There was the same treking across the Continent from one medical centre to another; the same alternation between attention to clinical matters and to pathology. But there were also significant differences. When John Thomson crossed the channel, he was already a mature and established practitioner. His sons and Carswell made their trips at the outsets of their careers; their European experience exerted a major influence upon the direction those careers subsequently took.

There was also a shift in the locus of pathological investigation. While John Thomson had been preoccupied with the preparations of morbid structures found in the museums of Europe, his acolytes spent more time studying pathology in the dead-room; Carswell in particular performed a huge number of autopsies in the French hospitals. It was from these immediate encounters with the relics of disease that they were to extract the pathological specimens and representations demanded by their master. Moreover, while there is a discontinuity between John Thomson's pathological and clinical observations, his sons and Carswell sought to correlate the two: to practise the true clinico-pathological method characteristic of the French.

All three mastered the most esoteric points of the techniques of physical examinations developed in France. They learned the use of the stethoscope together with the terminology Laennec had devised to characterize its findings.[67] Thus in a case of peripneumony at the Necker, Carswell noted that 'In this patient the râle crêpitant, was heard in the situation of the inferior lobe in the first degree and the noise of the respiration was totally wanting in that of the hepatized portion.'[68]

John Thomson, in contrast, developed a reputation for scepticism about the stethoscope. Although his biographer tried to repudiate this reproach, even he was obliged to acknowledge that Thomson had 'cautioned his students against an imprudent confidence in drawing inferences from stethoscopic signs'.[69] Thomson did refer to auscultation in his lectures on the institutes of medicine. He remarked that:

> Most of you must have heard of the instrument termed the Stethoscope, which was proposed by the late Professor Laennec[70] of Paris for facilitating the diagnosis of the Diseases of the Chest. The principle of the instrument is that it enables us to hear the noises produced by respiration, the Voice and the Motions of the heart; and as these noises differ in health & the different states of disease to which these organs are liable, it enables us to recognize the existence and nature of these diseases.[71]

In his discussion of respiration and circulation Thomson considered the stethoscope as a tool of *physiological* enquiry.

When as Professor of Pathology he came to discuss its clinical applications, Thomson's evaluation of auscultation was equivocal. He cast doubt on the novelty of the method maintaining that he had 'heard the purring sound of the arteries and Heart, 20 years before he saw Laennecs Treatise'. He also questioned the technique's potential: 'All Dr T. experience with the stethoscope has never enabled him to detect functional from organic

Disease of the Heart.'[72] When treating of pulmonary disease Thomson insisted that 'There is no certain knowledge of the existence of Tubercular matter in the lungs unless it is spit up.'[73] He did not even mention the application of the stethoscope in such cases. The general impression was that John Thomson – in contrast to his sons – never fully assimilated the technology and concepts of auscultation to his practice.

Although much was undoubtedly alien in the French metropolis, Thomson and Carswell may have been struck with similarities to their own town. 'Paris', wrote Thomas Hodgkin in 1822, 'in some respects bears more resemblance to Edinburgh than to London'. There were, for instance, the same common stairs on which several familes lived, as well as a similar

> inferior degree of cleanliness observable in the streets & also some of the customs of the lower orders. . . . As in Scotland the females take a considerable share of laborious outdoors employment. Both men and women carry burdens on their backs, the instrument which the men use for this purpose is completely Scotch.[74]

While in France William Thomson pursued a number of personal goals as well as furthering the objects his father had set. He took the opportunity of a protracted stay at the Hôtel-Dieu of Lyons to strengthen his credentials as a surgeon.[75] Carswell was more single-minded in his pursuit of Thomson's commission.

At the outset of the expedition Thomson regarded both Carswell and his son as subordinates who were to execute a plan of his design. In a letter to William Clift, the conservator of the Hunterian Museum in London, he described Carswell as 'an excellent Draughtsman and fond of the study of morbid anatomy'. Thomson asked Clift to 'point out to Mr Carswell some things for delineation which may be useful to me. We have got a good number of drawings from Mr William Hunter's Museum at Glasgow.'[76]

When his instruments showed signs of independence Thomson's response was sharp; he complained to William in July 1822 that

> I have not been able to learn by your packet of this morning whether you have received either of my last two letters nor whether the proposal of your going to Paris is to be carried out as I have recommended into execution or not. You have left me in utter ignorance of every thing Mr Carswell has done since he went to London and though I feel assured that he cannot have been idle still it would have been agreeable to me to have been informed either by you or by himself how he had been chiefly occupied[.][77]

Thomson went on to provide detailed instructions on how the two were to conduct their affairs while abroad. He was especially anxious that they take care to avoid conflict with another Scottish collector of pathology who might also be in Paris. William Cullen had proposed to the Royal College of Surgeons of Edinburgh that he should travel to France 'to make for them a museum of morbid anatomy'. Thomson was clearly concerned to avoid any appearance of competition with the representative of his 'patrons' while remaining determined to protect his own interests. 'If Cullen comes to Paris', he advised,

> I wish Carswell & you to give all the assistance in your power & while he gets a preparation for the college be you sure to get a description & drawing for me. In the way of preparations give up every thing to him that will not divide – but look sharply after every thing that is worth preserving for yourself.[78]

The direct link between what was to be done in France and Thomson's Edinburgh activities was highlighted when Thomson ordered his emissaries to 'put down for me' every thing that bore on diseases of the urinary and reproductive organs – the topics on which he proposed to lecture that winter.[79] In obedience to such instructions, the clinical and autopsy reports Carswell wrote in France were carefully correlated with the drawings he made; text and picture together would provide an effective teaching tool. In December 1822 Thomson suggested that William return to Edinburgh for a few months; as well as being able to assist in collecting materials at home for his father's teaching, 'your being with me during the time I am lecturing would let you see exactly what the delineations of diseases are of which I stand most in need. . . . Of course you will bring the drawings which Mr Carswell has already made along with you.'[80]

The pathological missions that Thomson organized conform in some respects to Bruno Latour's model of the structure and purpose of scientific expeditions. On this model, John Thomson's house on George Street became a centre of calculation to which specimens and inscriptions derived from the deadhouses of France were despatched.[81] The object, in Latour's terms, would have been to 'dominate' the phenomena of disease: to reduce their intractable multiplicity to a form which could be contained within Thomson's cabinet. His possession of such a resource would add to his reputation as a scientific authority. But the pathological allies that Thomson had assembled were put to more direct uses. These pictures and preparations were to be Thomson's assistants in the lecture room; the acclaim that they attracted in this setting would, in turn, strengthen his claims to academic advancement.

Within a few months of Carswell's arrival in France, however, the enterprise met with an unexpected check. When drawings were sent to Britain a punitive customs charge was levied upon them. Thomson invoked the aid of John Allen who in turn referred the matter to Sir Henry Halford.[82] When

Halford brought Thomson's grievance to the attention of the Chancellor of the Exchequer, he received an unsympathetic response. The government was prepared to waive the import duty on the drawings only if Thomson were to bequeath them to the University of Edinburgh after his death.

This suggestion brought an indignant reply from Allen: he declared that 'there is not . . . another country in Europe where such an undertaking as Dr Thomson's would not have received from its Government the slight and moderate encouragement he has solicited'. He expatiated upon the value of illustrations of disease to the student, maintaining that they were of far greater educational value than 'common anatomical preparations'. While the use of such illustrations was perhaps sufficiently well known in the elucidation of external disease, Thomson had taken the device a stage further:

> The drawings of Dr Th. which I have seen in E$^{dn.}$ contain not only an infinite variety of cutaneous diseases . . . but accurate & minute representations of the changes of structure in internal parts, delineated with the most perfect fidelity & coloured with the greatest carefulness.[83]

Allen dwelt upon the injustice of the government's proposal. It amounted to nothing less than an attack on the property rights of a private teacher for the benefit of a public institution. To propose to

> Dr Thomson, as a return for the remission of the Custom House duties, to divest himself of a property of so much value, acquired at a very considerable expence, and to transfer it to the University of Edinburgh, which has never thought of such a collection nor ever contributed a farthing to its formation, is fit only to be compared to a Clergyman offering a remission of tithes to his parishioners on condition that in return he should have the reversion of their Estates.

Should Thomson reject this proposal and the government insist on collecting the duty, the effect would be 'to put a stop to any further collections abroad'.[84]

The outcome of Allen's plea is not known. Its success may, however, be inferred from the fact that Thomson did not desist from the project: Carswell continued his work as Thomson's agent in France until 1826. Ultimately, the collection amounted to some 2,400 illustrations. It was first used in connection with Thomson's extramural lectures on the practice of physic and then for teaching general pathology in the university.[85]

Thomson's collection of illustrations attained a certain notoriety among both students and medical teachers in Edinburgh. A pamphlet of 1834 remarked – apropos of the creation of the chair of general pathology – that 'Even as a reward for having collected a valuable set of drawings, illustrative of diseased action, or for his consistent conduct as a Whig partizan, few would have objected to the appointment.'[86] When the question of the abolition of the chair arose, however, Thomson's antagonists sought to make polemical use of his favoured pedagogic technology. William Pulteney Alison argued:

> That the idea of General Pathology entertained by Dr Thomson sen., cannot be very different from mine, seems to me to be sufficiently proved by the fact, that the same extensive collection of drawings which he has used to illustrate his lectures on that subject had been previously used by him, with equally good effect, to illustrate his lectures on the Practice of Medicine.[87]

In other words, pathology was best taught as part of the practice of medicine rather than as a separate course of study.

James Syme incorporated Thomson's reliance on illustrations in his teaching into a much stronger attack upon the contention that general pathology was best taught as a separate subject. Syme argued that pathology should be part of the remit of the professors of the practice of medicine and of surgery; these chairs 'are universally admitted to require practical men for their occupants'. These professors were acknowledged to require something more than mere 'verbal knowledge of the things they profess to teach'. On the other hand,

> A Professor of General Pathology . . . need not be a practical man. He may be merely a man of respectable talents and application, well supplied with modern French books, and coloured delineations of morbid appearances, with the assistance of which he may not only appear to others, but even persuade himself, that he is truly acquainted with the subjects of his study.

Exposure to pedagogy of this sort must have a detrimental effect on the education of medical practitioners:

> the student would receive his first impressions of the things in which he is to be instructed from a source ever-varying in its doctrines with the fashion of the day. . . . Early impressions are not easily erased, and the very vagueness of their nature, if established by general statements and the exhibition of drawings, instead of the objects themselves, would still farther oppose their eradication, in order to make for those required in teaching the sound principles of medical and surgical practice. In illustration of this position, I beg to state that, in my deliberate opinion, a moderately diligent perusal of the Treatise on Carcinoma by the Professor of Pathological Anatomy in the

> University College, would fortify any student of ordinary talents against the most lucid and impressive explanation of no small part of a systematic surgical course.[88]

This professor of pathological anatomy was none other than Thomson's protégé, Robert Carswell.

While William Thomson returned to Britain in 1824, Carswell remained in France for several more years. From being John Thomson's instrument he gradually developed an identity and programme of his own; this was, however, in many ways an extension of Thomson's original design. He continued with the study of pathology, but now with a view to his own future career; he opened negotiations in December 1827 with the University of London for the creation of a new chair of pathological anatomy for himself.[89]

Carswell took over from Thomson the notion of coloured illustrations of disease as a pedagogic tool crucial to the success of the new course. He begged permission from the Council of London University to remain in Paris for two more years while he constructed this resource: 'It is by means of a sufficient number and a good choice of delineations that I can hope to simplify the study and communicate a knowledge of the material conditions of diseases, and thereby obtain the attendance of students on my lectures.'[90]

Carswell showed a keen awareness of the need to provide some such incentive to draw students to a course not recognized by any licensing body. Illustrations might also serve to persuade senior medical men of the interest and importance of the subject. He told Thomson in 1831 that

> I have made above a thousand delineations and have just got them arranged and hung up in one of the Theatres of the University not only to enable me to prepare my Lectures for the course which I *intend* to give next winter; but to give a full view of them to those gentlemen of the profession who may have the curiosity to come & see them. I called on Sir Jas. Macgregor t'other day. . . . He has promised to come & see them. I have also visited the Presidents of the College of Physicians & Surgeons & of the Apothecaries Company, and intend to write also to the Editors of Medical Journals and other persons of note. I have thought this the best plan I could adopt to give publicity to the subject, and to furnish me with an opportunity of demonstrating the utility of coloured representations of disease in the study of Pathological Anatomy.[91]

The Thomsons also regarded the illustrations they had accumulated as a means of selling their courses. The placards advertising the lectures they gave in 1820s featured this attraction. When in 1830 William Thomson took sole charge of the practice of physic course the advertisement noted that

> In conducting this Course, Mr Thomson will have an opportunity of illustrating the Morbid Alterations of Structure produced by Disease in the different Textures and Organs of the Human Body, by the extensive series of Coloured Delineations collected by his Father.[92]

When he became professor of medicine in Glasgow, Thomson took the illustrations with him. Despite the earlier attentions of the Exchequer, the collection remained an asset of the Thomson family.[93]

The liberal and philosophic physician

By 1820 John Thomson had virtually abandoned the practice of surgery although he still participated occasionally in surgical consultations. He had redefined himself as a physician; this identity was a prerequisite if he was to succeed in his ambition to become a professor of medicine in the university. Conversely, if he had obtained one of these posts, his standing as one of the leading medical practitioners in Edinburgh would have been secure. The failure of Thomson's attempts upon the chairs of the practice and institutes of medicine in 1821 has been outlined above.

His reaction to this setback was to disencumber himself of the two surgical chairs he had occupied and to commence once more as a private lecturer. In conjunction with William Thomson he began to teach the theory and practice of medicine at his house on George Street. In effect, the Thomsons set themselves up as a rival medical school in direct competition with the new incumbents of the university chairs. According to Charles Williams, who studied medicine in Edinburgh in the 1820s, this move met with considerable success. 'The inefficiency of the Chair of the Practice of Medicine in the College', he recalled, ' drove many students to the lectures of Dr John Thomson in the extra-academical school.' Williams added that Thomson's lectures 'were attractive, not only by their scientific tone, and from his earnestness and eloquence, but also through the illustrations of disease which they exhibited, in numerous coloured drawings of morbid anatomy. . . . These gave me the first insight into the appearances presented by the results of disease'.[94]

The George Street establishment can be considered not merely as an extramural rival but as a Whig opposition to the Tory academic regime. Just as Thomson's exclusion from the medical faculty was a matter of factional discrimination, so his response to that rebuff was replete with political meaning. The partisan aspect of his pedagogy was apparent in Thomson's choice of role-model: 'In discharging the duties of a public teacher', he declared,

> it will be my endeavour constantly to be guided by the sentiments expounded in regard to these duties by one who from the admirable

> manner in which he executed them for a long series of years must be acknowledged to be well acquainted with their nature – one in whose recent death the republic of Letters, & Philosophy has lost one of its brightest ornaments[.][95]

This paragon was the Whig Professor of Moral Philosophy, Dugald Stewart. The pedagogic principles that Stewart had expounded amounted to a form of intellectual liberalism. The 'public teacher' was not to seek to inculcate some dogmatic system, but to provide his students with the means to exercise their own judgements. The acquirement of this 'philosophic spirit' was the true end of the education of gentlemen.

Thomson sought to emulate these tenets chiefly in his course on the institutes or theory of medicine. This portion of the teaching at George Street was taken over by William Thomson after the 1826–7 session;[96] the manuscript notes are, however, predominantly in the father's hand with occasional emendations by the son. John Thomson should therefore be considered the author of the opinions expounded in those lectures.

In his introductory discourse Thomson explained the nature of the institutes of medicine along with its relations to other departments of medical knowledge. He adopted Cullen's tripartite classification of the subject maintaining that

> The Institutes of Medicine . . . consist of three Departments, the first relating to Health, which is termed Physiology, the 2nd relating to Disease, which is termed General Pathology & the 3d relating to remedies or mode of cure which is termed General Therapeutics.[97]

It was a matter of great moment to Thomson to establish that the first and second of these departments were of such extent that they must be taught separately. The self-sufficiency of general pathology was to be one of his chief justifications for his call for the creation of a new chair devoted to its cultivation. The lectures on the institutes that Thomson gave in the 1820s were chiefly concerned with physiology; pathology was reserved for a separate course on morbid anatomy.

He defined physiology as 'The department of Medical Science which investigates the laws of the different functions, both corporeal and mental, of the human economy in the state of health'.[98] In its identification of physiology as the science of the body in health this definition was unexceptional. Thomson's inclusion of *mental* phenomena within its ambit was, however, more remarkable. John Allen, when he planned his course in the 1790s, took great care to distinguish the study of the functions of the body – which was the province of physiology – from the investigation of the operations of the mind – which belonged to the metaphysician. Thomson, however, insisted on eliding the distinction. This was a potentially radical and provocative move. In France at the turn of the nineteenth century the claim that the physical and the moral formed two aspects of the same field had been used by ideologues like Cabanis (with whose writings Thomson was familiar) to justify a monistic concept of human nature. On this view, physiology was the true science of man; and those who cultivated it were entitled to take their place in society as a new priesthood.[99]

Thomson had no sympathy for monism; nor did he entertain such extravagant notions of the proper social role of medicine. His aim was not to reduce the study of mind to a branch of physiology, but to show that metaphysics formed a necessary part of the education of an enlightened medical practitioner. He thus adopted and adapted to medical education Stewart's axiom that a grounding in metaphysics was a prerequisite for the proper cultivation of the intellect (see chapter 1).

The model of the ideal practitioner with which Thomson operated owed less to French notions of medical bureaucracy than to native Scottish traditions of the attainments expected of a well-educated physician. Thomson in 1824 quoted John Gregory's assertion that

> besides the possession of a certain degree of knowledge of the Anatomical structure and Chemical composition of the human body, – of the uses of its different parts, and of the various organic functions which these parts perform – there is required also, on the part of the student and practitioner of medicine, an acquaintance with the Sensorial, Intellectual and Moral faculties with which man is endowed, with the reciprocal influences of his corporeal and mental faculties upon one another, – and with the changes to which, in the progress of health and disease, these faculties are subject. But how . . . is this knowledge to be obtained, unless by the study of Logic and of Moral Philosophy?[100]

The sum of these attainments distinguished the educated practitioner from the mass of empirics and quacks who also vied for the patronage of the public.

In his lectures on the institutes of medicine Thomson set out the bases for his conviction that 'the study of the Philosophy of the Human Mind has strong claims of the attention of those who intend to study Medicine as a science, or to practise it as a liberal art'. First, the medical student could derive certain general advantages from metaphysics: 'the Faculties of the Understanding are instruments which all men employ, and . . . it is impossible to employ them to the best advantage without a previous knowledge of their nature'. The science of mind possessed, however, a special call upon the attention of the medical man, 'because a most important and difficult branch of his duties is the treatment of those aberrations of the Mental faculties which form perhaps the most afflicting because the most humiliating class of diseases, to which Mankind is exposed'.[101]

For these reasons Thomson felt justified to 'introduce in this course a portion of what generally enters into courses of Metaphysics'. Early in his lectures he set out certain methodological principles which regulated all scientific endeavour. He insisted in particular upon the need for a sound understanding of the nature of cause and effect to those engaged in any 'philosophical Enquiry;' here the relevance of metaphysics was obvious:

> It is to Metaphysicians of comparatively modern date that we are indebted for having distinctly pointed out what import should be attached to those terms of Cause & Effect as employed in philosophical language; and those who know how much time has in consequence of misconception on this subject, been wasted in speculative enquiries that from their nature are beyond the reach of human intellect, will best appreciate the services of those who by establishing the accurate signification of these terms have distinctly defined the proper objects and limits of philosophical investigation.[102]

These metaphysicians had shown that the use of the terms cause and effect properly signified no more than that the occurrence of one event was invariably succeeded by the occurrence of another. It was impossible to go further and impute some necessary connection between the two. The recognition of these truths had important consequences for natural philosophy:

> To detect the occurrence of each intervening phenomenon, and to trace their influence in the production of particular events are undoubtedly legitimate objects of philosophical enquiry. But to suppose that when we have detected them we have advanced one step towards the solution of the question why in the given circumstances a particular phenomenon occurs rather than another – that we have discovered the chains which Nature makes use of to bind together her several operations is totally to misconceive the nature of the acquisitions we have made and of the faculties with which we have been endowed.[103]

On a slip of paper inserted into the notes Thomson acknowledged the source of this concept of causation: 'We could not foretel a single sequence. *D. Hume.*' His chief debt was, however, to the Scottish philosophers who sought to correct what they saw as the sceptical excesses of Hume's philosophy. Thomson described them as the 'champions who stood forth in Scotland to vindicate the authority of intuitive truths'.[104]

Thomson's lectures on the faculties of the human mind were little more than a recapitulation of the ideas of these 'common sense' philosophers. He had clearly studied Thomas Reid's *Essays* closely and adopted his classification of the emotions.[105] Thomson's chief debt was, however, to the writings of

Dugald Stewart: much of his metaphysical teaching consisted merely of lengthy quotations from the *Elements of the Philosophy of the Human Mind*.[106]

Thomson shared Stewart's hostility to any attempt to identify a physical basis for mental processes. Although he placed his discussion of the mental faculties in the section of the course that considered the nervous system, Thomson maintained that the relation between mind and brain was inscrutable. He rejected all attempts to hypothesize a material basis for memory or to suggest that intellectual faculties were represented in the brain.[107]

Just as there was a categorical boundary between the mental and the physical so there was an insuperable boundary between the human and animal. While he allowed that animals did have certain mental faculties in common with man – thus making possible a 'comparative metaphysics'[108] – Thomson followed Stewart in maintaining that humans possessed certain unique attributes. In particular, 'The boundary between the animal & the rational nature . . . is distinctly and strongly drawn by the capacity of artificial language, which none of the brutes possess even in the lowest degree.'[109]

Thomson thus aligned himself with a philosophy that eschewed any hint of controversial and heterodox views on human nature. His was a polite and respectable system of mental science free from any imputation of materialism, just as his politics – though mildly reformist – showed no real radicalism. The Whiggery of the George Street school was of the staid, conservative variety associated with the name of Dugald Stewart.

In other respects, however, Thomson's course on the institutes of medicine was innovatory. He revealed an extensive knowledge of recent work in French and German science and presented the results of these researches and speculations to his class. This teaching provided Edinburgh students with an early opportunity to become acquainted with the ideas of such major continental figures as Jean Baptiste Lamarck and Gottfried Treviranus who in the early nineteenth century were engaged in elaborating a new science of 'biology'.[110]

This science strove to identify the essential characteristics of living beings and to define the terms of a discourse devoted to the explication of vitality. Thomson accordingly devoted much time in his lectures to an exposition of the principles of 'general physiology' – the study of the most fundamental phenomena of life. He offered various definitions of life drawn from the authors he used as sources. On occasion, he approximated to Cuvier's concept of the living body as a 'tourbillon': 'Life', Thomson maintained, 'consists in the faculty which certain corporeal combinations have of continuing for a time under a determinate form.'[111] He also echoed the holistic aspect of Cuvier's concept of the living body when he argued that:

> The organized body exists only as a whole. All the parts of which it is composed are mutually dependant [*sic*] on one another and they cannot be separated from one another without a cessation of their existence as a living [being?] and a destruction of the whole.[112]

In his adoption of the Cuvierian concept of the organism, as in other respects, Thomson followed John Allen's precedent. When he left Edinburgh Allen donated the notes he had prepared for his lectures to Thomson who referred to them at several points in his course. But there were aspects of Thomson's concept of general physiology which were either only rudimentary or wholly lacking in Allen. In particular, Thomson showed a much greater awareness of the need for a *comparative* approach to the elucidation of physiological questions.

If vital processes were to be fully understood, it was necessary to study them in their most basic manifestation; for example, 'in order to ascertain whether any physical powers are essential to living bodies in addition to those possessed by inorganic bodies, we must examine living bodies under the most simple form in which they occur'.[113] Since many vital processes were most rudimentary in plants, Thomson therefore felt it necessary to give his students a grounding in vegetable physiology.[114]

Once the study of life was detached from that of any particular organism, certain important principles became clear. The first of these was the priority of function over structure. Thus infusoria and polyps 'must be considered as composed of elementary animal texture possessing all the properties which we see in separate textures & distinct parts in higher animals'.[115] The organs that performed these functions in man emerged through a process of gradual elaboration in the animal series. Circulation, for instance, was an operation common to all animals; but 'we find no organ analogous to a heart in Microscopic animalcules or in Zoophites'. Annelids were furnished with a contractile tube through which fluid was propelled. But the 'Crustacea . . . is the first class in w^{h} we find a true heart'. Thomson observed that this development was correlated with other structural novelties: it was

> remarkable that at that part of the scale of animals in which we first find animals to possess a distinct heart we also observe a liver or analogous organ and a more perfect mode of respiration; for all those animals which possess a heart breathe either by means of lungs or gills which may generally be described as organs so constituted as that the blood that passes through them is exposed to the atmospherical air.[116]

Thomson therefore expounded in his lectures the notion of a scale of living beings which displayed a clear progression whereby simpler passed imperceptibly into more elaborate organisms. Despite his numerous references to Lamarck, however, he never hinted at the possibility of transformism – indeed, Thomson studiously ignored this aspect of Lamarck's thought. Nor is there any hint of the influence of the environment in generating organic change, or of Lamarck's doctrine of spontaneous generation. Thomson's chain of being remained an unexplained datum.

These silences were significant. They signalled the crucial distinction between Thomson's biology and the Lamarckianism of another extramural lecturer, Robert E. Grant. In his lectures and writings Grant emphasized the transformist aspects of Lamarck's work.[117] Speculations of this ilk possessed grave theological implications: in particular, they threatened the notion of a fixed permanent design and of man's special status within that scheme.[118] Lamarck, for example, viewed mental faculties merely as physiological functions which progressively emerged in the course of evolution.[119] Such doctrines were incompatible with Thomson's stated views on human nature. In particular, they could not be reconciled with his commitment to the existence of unique human intellectual attributes and to the independence of mind of bodily organization.

He was also unlikely to be sympathetic to the radical political connotations that Lamarckianism acquired in early nineteenth-century Britain.[120] He presented a safe, carefully censored version of Lamarck's ideas which was unlikely to offend religious sensibilities or to foster rumours promulgated by his enemies that he was an advocate of 'extreme opinions even in favour of popular rights'.[121]

Thomson also distanced himself, however, from the physiological views favoured by the other political extreme. He was sceptical to the point of being contemptuous of the promiscuous use some made of the term 'vital principle'. He remarked that

> we thrust in this poor jaded vital principle wherever we are ashamed to confess our ignorance – Some have attempted to defend this by saying that we only employ it as the most general law applicable to the changes of living bodies as we do gravitation repulsion &c in Chemistry & Mechanics but how is it that we should only have one general principle as the cause of those living actions so much more diversified and inexplicable than those of Chemistry & Mechanics in which several have been inserted[?][122]

This was an undisguised attack upon the use of the term vital principle made by William Pulteney Alison in his lectures as professor of the institutes of medicine.[123]

Such trimming was typically Whig. It was an aspect of a discourse which took pride in steering a course between radicalism on the one hand and reaction on the other. The school of medicine over which Thomson presided in the 1820s was safe when compared to the doctrines expounded by such private lecturers as Grant or Robert Knox.[124] At the same time it was not afraid to criticize the orthodoxies professed in the College. It was a respectable, if not entirely loyal, opposition that might aspire eventually to become the ruling academic party.

The able and experienced practitioner

Compared to the wealth of material available on John Thomson's teaching, there is relatively little record of his activities as a medical practitioner. What there is consists chiefly of correspondence with patients and with other practitioners and dates from the period after 1820. By this date Thomson was a senior and successful member of the medical profession in Edinburgh. A measure of his success can be gleaned from his appointment books.[125] He also enjoyed a national reputation as an accomplished practitioner: the London physician John Armstrong in 1825 described Thomson as 'one of the ablest and most experienced medical gentlemen in this or any other country'.[126]

He had by this time largely abandoned surgery and identified himself primarily as a physician. Thus around 1825 Thomson was the medical adviser to a patient suffering from progressive paralysis while John Lizars acted as surgeon in the case.[127] Thomson was, however, still occasionally consulted on surgical matters both by patients and by colleagues. For example, in October 1829, a Cramond practitioner wrote to him about

> a patient three months old who had scrotal hernia which was removed by a few weeks application of a trap – within the last 10 days a tumour has appeared . . . the exact nature of which puzzles me a great deal – and I have therefore requested the childs mother . . . to take him to town for your advice.[128]

Even in 1834 Thomson was still asked to take part in the management of a surgical case. When the publisher William Blackwood was afflicted with a pendulous tumour, Thomson was involved in a consultation with Robert Liston and James Syme on how best to remove the growth. The case illustrates how delicate the business of consultation could be: Liston stormed from the sick room because he felt that his opinion had been ignored and that Thomson had slighted his professional character in the patient's hearing.[129]

Thomson's caseload was wide and varied showing no evidence of any particular bias or specialization. In 1827 he treated patients suffering from asthma, intestinal worms, hernia, and a gynaecological complaint – as well as trying to assist a young man afflicted with the 'dreadful malady' of drunkenness.[130] Occasionally, however, individuals did seek Thomson out because of his reputation in a particular field; his known interest in the treatment of syphilis gained him at least one patient.[131]

As a pedagogue Thomson set out clear principles of therapeutics. He presented himself as a proponent of the antiphlogistic method; but he tended to a minimalist, expectant approach to the treatment of disease. He recommended the use of only a small number of remedies, reminding his students

> of those salutary changes which nature, aided by diet and regimen, often accomplishes, but which are usually ascribed by the ignorant to the operation of the medicines that have been administered during the time that those natural and salutary changes, by which diseases are, in fact, ultimately cured or relieved, have been going on in the constitution.[132]

This was an extension of the Hunterian doctrine Thomson had adopted in his surgical lectures where he maintained that 'the mechanical and chemical means which the Surgeon employs in this and in every other exercise of his art, are merely subsidiary to the healing process of nature'.[133] It also echoed Dugald Stewart's encomium to the 'wisdom of nature' (see chapter 2, p. 71): indeed Thomson's therapeutics can be seen as a practical endorsement of a philosophy which extolled the self-sufficiency and competence of the body. He extended this doctrine even to diseases where medical intervention was usually considered as necessary to achieve a cure. In 1817 Andrew Duncan junior noted that

> A very respectable surgeon [i.e. Thomson], who has the best means of determining practical questions, has reported, that so many cases of venereal ulcers, and venereal sore throats, have got well without a grain of mercury, that he considers the human constitution, as possessing natural powers adequate to the cure of a disease, in which it was believed to be fully ascertained that nature was utterly insufficient. These reports, from so respectable a man, have staggered many physicians, have produced belief in a few persons, and are not credited by others[.][134]

It was, therefore, in Thomson's view a fundamental principle of medical practice to secure 'fair play to nature'.[135] Such a therapeutic strategy could, however, be successfully conducted only by rational and not by purely empirical practitioners: it was predicated upon a knowledge of the workings of nature as exposed by the sciences of physiology and pathology.

But at least as important to professional success as these intellectual attainments was the moral character of the physician. Thomson was praised for his manner with patients: 'His intercourse with the sick', an obituarist recalled,

> was singularly agreeable, bringing into exercise not only the vigour of his understanding but the kindly dispositions of his heart. The interest which he manifestly took in the individual circumstances of his patients, speedily inspired them with the confidence that their ailments were duly considered, and understood as far as science and skill would allow; and that nothing would be neglected that could contribute to their cure or relief.[136]

There is confirmation in Thomson's correspondence that he did cultivate close social relations with some of his patients. One elderly lady wrote to him from Newcastle-upon-Tync in 1833 'to express my grateful sense of your kindness and Consideration of me last Winter, as [much?] as to assure you, of the great benefit I have derived from your valuable Advice'. The regime Thomson had recommended included 'ambling about during the Summer upon a Donkey'. The letter concludes, 'if I should visit Edin^r again, I shall certainly have the pleasure of waiting upon you, and perhaps showing you that I am the stout old woman you predicted I should be'.[137]

Thomson's practice encompassed all strata of the social hierarchy. In 1822 Margaret Thomson reported that her husband had been summoned to Castle Mingies near Dunkeld

> To visit Sir Neil Mingies who has been for some months labouring under the effects of a severe compound fracture in the limb . . . your fathers being called was at the suggestion of the attending surgeon on the spot whom there had been an attempt to find wrong by some of the Perth surgeons – who suggested an operation against his opinion. This difference of opinion ended very agreeably for the Patient as well as for your father by his finding no necessity for an amputation, and by his relieving him of a piece of dead bone which was the cause of the irritation.[138]

Upon his return to Edinburgh Thomson attended another case which 'communicated not less satisfaction though in an inferior class of society'. A young man

> a journeyman Shoemaker had swallowed a half crown and after having it 24 hours down his throat his friends came and entreated your father to visit him. He went taking Turner with him, and found him in great uneasiness and his friends around him weeping and in great distress – Your Father first put down a *probos* and felt it just at the orifice of the stomach, and then hooked it and on the first effort got it up to his gullet, and on a second turned it into his mouth to the great joy of all round and much to his own satisfaction – It happened the day he came home – so that in these two days he had the pleasure to save one mans leg, and anothers life.[139]

Although he treated both aristocrats and artisans, Thomson's private patients were mostly drawn from among his peers in Edinburgh society: they were clergymen, accountants, lawyers, and the members of the families of such men. This shared status facilitated social familiarity; patients sometimes indicated in their letters that they were acquainted with Thomson's wife and sons and so had personal as well as professinal links with him.

An anonymous letter of 1817 alleged that Thomson's clientele showed a pronounced political bias: he was alleged to have 'a practice among the Jacobins here equal to £2000'.[140] Given that political differences did during this period impinge upon all forms of social interaction, it may well be that Thomson's patients, as well as his friends, were drawn from among those of a Whig persuasion. But there are only a few hints of such an elective affinity in his correspondence. Thomson attended Dugald Stewart during his last illness and forwarded news of his condition to John Allen for transmission to Lauderdale.[141] There are also letters to Thomson from Charles Findlater written in 1832 in which discussion of the patient's health is accompanied by references to the passage of the Reform Bill and complaints about the Toryism of the established Scottish clergy.[142]

The main outlines of Thomson's professional persona correspond with notions of the typical eighteenth-century polite physician. His attention to the patient as a whole person, rather than merely the embodiment of a disease process, conforms, for instance, to Jewson's model of a practitioner of 'bed-side medicine'.[143] Thomson's patients, moreover, occasionally demonstrated the familiarity with medical knowledge that according to Jewson permitted them to interact on an equal footing with their medical advisers.[144]

Despite the overt modernism of his medical theory Thomson emerges therefore as a traditional medical practitioner; he continued, for instance, to teach a version of the doctrine of the four humours to his pathology class.[145] His ability to conceptualize disease in the classroom or deadhouse as a lesion of the constituent tissues of the body had no apparent impact upon his interactions with his private patients. This impression is strengthened by the fact that he continued the eighteenth-century practice of offering diagnoses by post.[146] When Georgina Fox fell ill, Thomson forwarded a long written opinion on her case to John Allen without laying eyes – still less hands – on the patient (see appendix A).

There were, however, ways in which Thomson's activities as a teacher and pathologist did intersect with his practice. His academic reputation was responsible for some of the consultations which Thomson received. In the 1829 case of scrotal hernia mentioned above he was addressed as 'John Thomson, Professor of Pathology'. This was technically incorrect; but it does reveal the light in which the practitioner seeking the consultation viewed Thomson. In the same year Thomson was asked to visit

> Mrs Wilson Windmill Lane – since you saw her last a tumor on the course of the Carotid has appeared, the nature of which I am at a loss to determine, whether aneurismal or an enlarged Gland receiving its pulsation from the Artery, if the former I fear it will soon be all over with her.[147]

The implication was that Thomson possessed special knowledge of pathological anatomy that might assist in making a differential diagnosis.

Patients and their families too were aware of Thomson's academic status; one wrote in 1831 to congratulate him 'with all my heart on your appointment to a professorship in the University which I am sure you must fill with great benefit to the profession and credit to yourself'.[148]

The network of contacts among local practitioners forged by such consultations could also provide opportunities to increase that knowledge. An East Linton doctor advised Thomson in April 1828 that 'The girl Aitchinson at Lynningham died this morning and as I have got permission to inspect the body tomorrow, I should be happy if your Son or any of your friends, could come and witness the dissection, as I know that you have a great interest in these cases.'[149] Thomson had therefore acquired among Edinburgh practitioners a reputation as a pathological consultant – an 'experienced dissector' whose opinion could elucidate doubtful post-mortem appearances.[150]

The consent of the patient's family to perform such inspections was required; and this was not always forthcoming. When Mrs Wilson died, the practitioner who had consulted Thomson 'tried as much as I could to get permission to examine, but without success their feelings would not allow them'.[151] Paradoxically, the personal relationship that Thomson developed with some of his patients could serve to overcome such resistance. When one of these died a relative wrote to regret that Thomson had not been present

> because his only confidence in medical advice rested on you and altho. I believe every thing was done by those Gentlemen who attended him, that medical aid could do – yet it would have been more desirable to have had the assistance of one – had he had the power of attendance – he would have called upon himself.

Permission to open the body was given and Thomson invited to attend the last medical rite.[152] In this instance, consent to autopsy constituted a final homage from a patient's family to the personal and professional qualities of the attending physician. Far from contradicting the relationship of trust between patient and practitioner that had existed in life by reifying him in death, post-mortem examination appeared as its natural consummation.

Another token of Thomson's status as the leading pathologist in Edinburgh was the flow of parcels to his George Street address containing specimens forwarded by practitioners around the country. He formed the centre of a network for the communication of objects and ideas. Shortly after Christmas 1827, for instance, James Stenhouse of Dunfermline begged leave 'to send you a mamma which was cut out today by Mr Alexander Surgeon here – Perhaps you may find it worthy of notice.'[153] Charles Cheyne of Leith likewise despatched 'for examination (and a place in your museum if worthy of it) a specimen of scirrhus of the tongue removed today from the body of a poor woman who died yesterday'.[154]

Various motives can be suggested for this traffic in body parts. By seeking to establish a gift-relationship with Thomson these practitioners may have hoped to have placed him under an obligation to them which might in future redound to their professional interest. But these doctors also seemed eager to contribute their mite to a grand collective enterprise of which Thomson was the acknowledged director. However humble their station and mundane their practice, they might nevertheless add something to the stock of pathological knowledge. In 1822 Thomson sought to formalize these contacts by inviting selected practitioners to join a society dedicated to the cultivation of this science.[155]

Towards the end of his career there are signs that Thomson found it increasingly difficult to reconcile the competing demands on his time and energy of the different aspects of the compound professional role that he had sought to fill. He relied increasingly on substitutes to deliver his lectures while he was abroad visiting patients some of whom lived many miles from Edinburgh. It is, however, impossible to draw any simple distinction between his clinical, pedagogic and scientific concerns; this chapter has shown how the three were intertwined to form the texture of Thomson's professional identity. As age and infirmity took their toll Thomson was obliged to restrict his own activities in all these areas. He looked increasingly to his sons to perpetuate the political and professional aspirations to which he had devoted his life.

Appendix A

Edin^{r} Octob^{r} 4th 1819

Dear Allen

After studying attentively your description of Georgina's case I confess that I am not able to form a perfectly decided opinion with regard to its nature. I am inclined to believe that there is no organic affection, and that the greater part of the symptoms which have occurred have arisen from derangement of the Digestive and Biliary organs. The affection of the chest was certainly much to be dreaded but from it appearing to be on the decrease instead of increasing, and from her breathing being so easy I should hope that no positive mischief exists in her lungs.

The view I am disposed to take of Georgina's case is that her disease was originally Remittent fever which in young persons particularly if they retain any appetite for their food is often a disease of long duration and followed by emaciation and continued quickness of pulse. I have frequently seen it precede and appear to be kept up by sudden growth, and though you do not mention this as having occurred in Georgina yet I should not be surprized to find that her present ailments were connected with an addition to her stature – I attended very lately a young girl about her age in whom the symptoms were almost exactly those which you describe and although her fever has been double the length of Georgina and her pulse is even still remarkably quick I now consider her as convalescent – The state of the urine which you mention I conceive to be dependent upon the biliary derangement – A red tinge as if from blood I have frequently seen in cases of fever without any organic affection.

From your letter I perceive that there is but little for me to suggest on the subject of Georgina's food. I would certainly be inclined to continue the diet of milk and farinaceae in the forms and quantities that agree with and are agreeable to her. If the animal soup does not appear to have the effect of heating her there can be no objection to its forming with bread or rice the greater part of her dinner. But till the febrile state shall abate considerably I should be very cautious in allowing her any solid animal food – I do not know of any better medicine for keeping her bowels regular than Rhubarb and Magnesia or the Compound Rhubarb Pill. If notwithstanding their use the clayish colour of the stools should continue a dose of Calomel may be occasionally administered with perfect safety to her constitution.

I would avoid Narcotic and Nauseating remedies of all sorts and endeavour to procure a healthy state of the skin by the use of the warm bath. Care should be taken that the temperature is not too high nor the immersion too long continued as from each of these causes I have often seen the beneficial effects of warm bathing defeated. I would fain hope that the warm bathing will be found beneficial to the cough and in the progress of recovery that you will be able to convert it into a Tonic in the form of the tepid *douche*.

I throw out these suggestions the more readily that they are precisely the measures which I would be inclined to follow even if I had reason to suspect an affection of the lungs. I have only to add that in contemplating the possibility of such an affection I would avoid as much as possible the continued use of Mercurials, and should the cough continue or appear to increase I would make no scruple to apply one or more blisters to the chest.

I shall be anxious to hear from you that the cough and the febrile symptoms gradually decline. Mild nourishment will be found I am convinced the best restorative but your own observation and the experience of the Medical Attendants must direct the choice and administration of this.

I have only to repeat that I would abstain as much as possible from the use of Narcotic and Nauseating Medicines as they always disturb more or less the state of the Digestive and Biliary Organs and prevent by this our being able to perceive the real state of matters in many of the diseases in which they are employed.

Yours faithfully
John Thomson.
(BL Additional MS 52194 f. 131)

5

A Whig decline

The elder son

William Thomson was born in Edinburgh in July 1802. He was the second of John Thomson's sons by his first wife. William was at first intended for the law; but the death of his brother made him heir to the family's medical mantle. He therefore entered the university as a student of medicine. His medical studies seem, however, to have been rudimentary: he is known to have taken only anatomy, chemistry, practice of medicine, and possibly materia medica and clinical medicine in the university. He never satisfied the requirements for graduation and was eventually obliged, like his father, to purchase a MD from Aberdeen.[1]

After passing the 1821–2 session undertaking further studies in Glasgow, Thomson joined Robert Carswell in the first of their pathological forays to France (see chapter 4). As well as collecting specimens for his father's museum, Thomson took the opportunity to attend Laennec's lectures on pathology.[2]

He also travelled to the Netherlands, Germany, Austria and Italy in the company of other medical men. They toured through Europe at breakneck speed in the spring and summer of 1825: Utrecht merited a stay of one and a half days while Amsterdam detained them for three. The special object of Thomson's attention during this trip was the various methods of clinical teaching adopted in the centres through which they passed. At Leyden, Thomson complained, 'we did not see any hosp: the professor of clinical medicine was not inclined to shew his wards, it being a Saturday'.[3] In Liège, on the other hand, though they stayed only two hours, he was 'present at the clinical visit, which was conducted in a small ward, with a degree of quietness, almost approaching to secrecy, and followed by a clinical lecture in French, by which we were not much edified'.[4]

The tone of these remarks is typical of the self-assured and critical manner in which Thomson approached the efforts of the foreign professors whom he observed. Professor Nasse of Bonn was dismissed as 'a man of considerable reading and little judgment, [who] rests his opinion on very insufficient foundations and consequently changes them frequently'. Thomson conceded that Nasse possessed 'a considerable talent in lecturing and explaining'. But he added that 'His pupils warned me against receiving any of his published accounts of dissections as gospel: as he is very liable to deceive himself or to be deceived by others in these subjects.'[5]

Johann Lucas Schönlein of Würzburg came off somewhat better: he was described as 'rather a young man, of much zeal and intelligence who after having gone through the schools of the transcendental philosophy has returned to sound views on the road of experience'. Unfortunately, however, 'being placed alone and in the midst of his admiring pupils, he does not escape the injurious influence of which the possession of arbitrary power has on the mind'.[6] Even in the clinic Whig political maxims had their application.

More important than these peculiarities of personality were Schönlein's accomplishments as a clinician. Thomson noted Schönlein's claim to have 'established a diagnosis of *tubercles of the encephalon*: a fixed pain with heaviness in a part of the head, stupor, and finally frequent epileptic fits'. This diagnosis had been verified in several cases at autopsy.[7]

The organization of the clinical schools he visited also received Thomson's close attention. The medical clinic at Heidelberg was, in general, well conducted; but Thomson noted an important weakness in its plan. Almost all 'the patients admitted are men- and maidservants, *young adults* so that the pupils are familiarised only with the constitution of this time of life.'[8]

Thomson's special preoccupation with clinical teaching in European medical centres is explained by events nearer home. In 1826 a Royal Commission on the Universities of Scotland was to begin hearing evidence. In his testimony before the Commission John Thomson urged the creation of a new chair of clinical medicine in Edinburgh; the example of foreign universities provided much of the argumentative resources that Thomson deployed. In his observations in German clinics, as well as in his labours in French deadhouses, William was supplying the demands of his father's domestic campaigns.

After his second continental tour, William Thomson settled in Edinburgh late in 1825, and set about establishing his credentials as a surgeon. He was admitted to the Fellowship of the Royal College of Surgeons after submitting a dissertation on lithotomy[9] and secured a surgical appointment at the New Town Dispensary. These efforts to create an independent professional identity were, however, tempered by William's continued involvement in the family firm. He lectured on the institutes of medicine in 1826–7, as well as assisting his father in teaching the practice. As noted above, the degree of his tutelage is demonstrated by the fact that it was John Thomson who wrote most of the lectures that his son delivered at this time. William was, in effect, serving an apprenticeship as a medical teacher. As he grew more experienced, his father was prepared to allow him more responsibility; he nevertheless continued to control the trajectory of his son's career. Whatever William's own ambitions may have been, John Thomson had decided his destiny: he was to succeed him as a professor in the Faculty of Medicine in Edinburgh University.

The circumstances under which this ambition was frustrated have already been described (see chapter 3). Although William continued to teach the general pathology course until his father finally retired, both had realized that there was no possibility that he would ever occupy a university position in Edinburgh. He could, at most, hope to revert to lecturing in the extramural school.

In the course of the 1830s William had taken care to multiply his options. He followed his father's example by acquiring credentials as a physician: he took an MD from Aberdeen in 1831 and two years later became a Fellow of the Royal College of Physicians of Edinburgh. Finally, in 1840 he was appointed one of the physicians to the Royal Infirmary. These provisions supplied William with the foundations for a successful medical practice in the city; but they also served to strengthen his claims on academic opportunities elsewhere.

As early as 1827, John Thomson, in a bout of depression over prospects in Edinburgh, expressed the hope that in the aftermath of the Royal Commission on the Scottish universities new medical chairs might be created in Glasgow. 'I wish', he added, 'I could get one of them for William.'[10] After 1800 the medical school in Glasgow had emerged as a serious competitor to Edinburgh, not least because its graduation requirements were somewhat laxer. It might therefore provide an alternative site for an academic career.

William Thomson's chance finally came in 1840 when his prospects of advancement in Edinburgh had disappeared. He received a communication from John Badham, Professor of Medicine at Glasgow, 'expressing his willingness to resign his chair in the event of the Government agreeing to allow him to retain £300 a year out of the emoluments of the office'. These emoluments were considerable: the professor received a salary of £270, a free house, as well as class and graduation fees of around £350 a year.[11]

Thomson promptly wrote to the Lord Advocate seeking support for this proposition. Andrew, Lord Rutherfurd (1791–1854) was a veteran Edinburgh Whig and likely to be receptive to a plea from a member of the Thomson family.[12] As a further inducement, Thomson warned that if the arrangement were not agreed, there was a danger of the chair passing into less congenial hands. He reminded the Advocate that 'of the fourteen members of the Faculty or governing body of Glasgow College, the government cannot reckon more certainly than three friends'.[13] Thomson supplied a visual aid designed to impress this important point on Rutherfurd:

Faculty of the Glasgow College

	Principal Macfarlane	
	Professor Nichol +	
Crown patron	–	Davidson D
	–	Jeffray D
	–	Badham D
	–	Macturk
	–	Ramsay
	–	Lushington +?
	–	Ja. Thomson +
Senatus Academicus		Meikleham D
		Buchanan
		Fleming
		Gray
		(Divinity vacant)

Notes: + Liberal; D Acting by Deputy.[14]

Placing a Thomson in the Faculty would help to redress the balance. In a letter to James Oswald, Thomson laid still more stress on party considerations. Badham's terms must be accepted because otherwise the chair might pass either to his son or, 'as is supposed to be the object with certain superannuated professors in Glasgow College, in retaining their chairs, a successor attached to his own political party'. Thomson did not overlook the 'desireableness of having the Chair in question filled by a Teacher more competent for its arduous duties than Dr Badham can be expected ever again to be, and I believe I may add without scandal of greater professional zeal'. There was, however,

> another consideration to which I may advert, not certainly as a ground for countenancing any improper arrangement either in the way of resignation or appointment, but as an inducement to take some pains in effecting a proper arrangement, I mean, the desireableness for the advancement of liberal opinions and of improvements in the system of the Scottish Universities of the Chairs in the Faculty or governing body of Glasgow College, being almost exclusively occupied by gentlemen of Tory principles[.][15]

The government's response to Thomson's plea came in 1841 when a commission was issued appointing him Professor of Medicine in the University of Glasgow. The commission stipulated that

> whereas the Professor of Medicine in the University of Glasgow has hitherto given Lectures both on the Theory and the Practice of Physic

> and it may hereafter be deemed expedient that these branches of Medical Science should each be taught by a separate Professor and the duties of the Professor of Medicine subdivided nothing herein contained shall in any respect be held to prevent Her Majesty from naming an additional Professor for the Teaching of either of the Theory or of the Practice of Physic in the University of Glasgow[.][16]

This caveat harked back to extensive discussions during the hearings of the Royal Commission on Scottish Universities in 1827 on the advisability of separating the teaching of medical theory and practice in Glasgow. In his evidence Richard Millar, lecturer upon materia medica, had urged the creation of a separate chair of medical theory; as well as its academic advantages, such an innovation would, he argued, help to remedy a deficiency of physicians in the city.[17] Millar was a staunch Whig and something of a pariah within the university. His proposal was resisted by the Tory majority in the medical faculty. The Professor of Anatomy, James Jeffray, in particular, insisted that the teaching of theory and practice should be conjoined. To say that professors of medicine and surgery

> shall not be at liberty to treat either of the physiology or pathology of any part affected with disease, but that the one should confine himself to the shewing how this or that operation should be performed, and the other to the directing whether medicines should be given, would be to cut them off from all that is intellectual in their course of practical instruction.[18]

The commissioners none the less in their report of 1829 recommended that a new chair of the theory of medicine should be established in Glasgow; and in 1839 Andrew Buchanan (1798–1882) was appointed as the first incumbent. When he came to Glasgow Thomson was therefore able to confine his teaching to the practice of medicine on the Edinburgh model.

Thomson took an active part in university politics during his time in Glasgow. He was loyal to those who had appointed him – serving the interests of the Whig party in general and of Rutherfurd in particular. He kept the Advocate informed of political tendencies within the university and sought to further his interests: in 1848, for instance, Thomson orchestrated support for Rutherfurd's candidacy for the post of Rector of Glasgow University.[19]

Thomson also pursued an ideal of citizenship, taking an active part in the affairs of his new home city. He was a Director of both the Royal Infirmary and of the Gartnavel Lunatic Asylum and devoted much time to the affairs of both institutions. His chief concern, however, was the improvement of the university to which he now belonged. Thomson served for six years as Clerk to Faculty. His concerns went beyond the purely factional. He was not merely concerned to break the Tory grip upon the

Glasgow College, but also to abolish the corrupt practices associated with this regime. His aim was both to liberalize and to modernize the institution; to encourage the appointment of men of correct political opinions who could also be relied upon to reform and uplift the medical school.

William Thomson's early death from heart disease on 10 May 1852 meant that he did not see these plans come to fruition. The same cause was, however, from 1848 championed in Glasgow with great vigour by his younger brother.

The born professor

Allen Thomson was born on 2 April 1809 in Edinburgh. His mother was John Thomson's second wife, Margaret Millar. While his immediate roots were in the east, he thus possessed hereditary links with Glasgow. He owed his Christian name to his father's longstanding friend and ally, John Allen. The younger Thomson thus embodied in his person various strands of the history of the Whig party in Scotland at the turn of the nineteenth century.

Like his brother, after attending the High School, Allen in 1824 entered Edinburgh University. Unlike William, there was never any question but that he would pursue a career in medicine. From the first, moreover, his education was tailored towards qualifying him to enter the elite of the profession. Between 1825 and 1830 Allen Thomson passed through the courses requisite for graduation. In 1830 he presented an MD thesis titled *De evolutione cordis in animalibus vertebratis.* This he illustrated himself, demonstrating his accomplishments as an artist. Even at this early date he already displayed a bent for theoretical rather than practical subjects and, in particular, for what was to be his chief passion – embryology. While a student Thomson enjoyed the honour of being President of the Royal Medical Society. He also took an active part in the proceedings of the Plinian Society, a student association devoted to the pursuit of natural history. The minutes of the Plinian record Thomson as one of six members who on 26 June 1827

> met at the Botanic Garden and walked towards the sea shore at Newhaven, from this they proceeded up the shore of the Firth of Forth as far as Cramond, one party exploring the recesses of the woods of Granton, while another employed themselves on the shore collecting shells and seaplants.[20]

Thomson formed part of the latter contingent.

Before graduating Thomson made his first professional visit to the Continent spending several months in Paris. There he contributed to his father's great project of pathological enquiry by taking part in dissections and recording the appearances by means of drawings. Allen was never, however, as deeply involved in this undertaking as was his brother and

Carswell; most of his time was spent in the pursuit of his own interests. He attended Magendie's lectures on physiology, Dulong's on physics, Andral's on hygiene, and Blainville's on zoology. He also followed the medical clinic of A.F. Chomel at the Charité.[21]

In 1831 Thomson became a Fellow of the Royal College of Surgeons in Edinburgh, but only to qualify himself to lecture in the extramural school. In contrast to his father and brother he never displayed any desire to be a surgeon. Encouraged by John Thomson, he had already decided upon a career as a teacher of medical science. To this end he toured the schools and museums of Europe in 1831 collecting specimens and illustrations to use in his projected course.

Thomson was accompanied on this journey by William Sharpey (1802-80) a former student of his father. On their return to Edinburgh they formed a teaching partnership that lasted until 1836. While Sharpey lectured on anatomy Thomson confined himself to physiology. He did, however, assist Sharpey with the anatomical demonstrations in order to familarize himself with this branch of medical education.

The smooth progress of Thomson's academic career was interrupted in 1836 by a bout of bad health that forced him to leave Edinburgh. Just as John Allen had sought refuge in the Holland household, so his namesake found temporary shelter in the employ of another Whig magnate – John Russell, sixth Duke of Bedford.

Russells and rustics

The arrangement had advantages for both parties. It provided the Russells – and especially the valetudinarian Duke – with a qualified practitioner on their travels. On the other hand, his new position removed Thomson from the reek of Edinburgh and took him to more salubrious climes. There were, however, also drawbacks to doctoring a duke.

Above all, there was the problem of Thomson's authority as a practitioner over his patients. He was, if not quite an employee, then certainly a client of the Russell household. As patrons his patients expected to have a large say in the direction of their cases; they were, moreover, opinionated in medical matters and loath to concede Thomson's superior diagnostic and therapeutic expertise.[22] The fact that Thomson was still a young man with limited clinical experience made these difficulties the more acute.

On several occasions he felt the need to appeal to his father for advice. In a letter of 28 June 1836 from Woburn Abbey he revealed that the Duke 'had a distinct paralytic attack proceeding from a cerebral affection. . . . He has a tendency of blood to the head'. Although he had been briefed on the previous management of the case by the Duke's former attendant, Thomson admitted that 'I should like very much if you find time that you could give me a few hints about the treatment'. The problem was as much a managerial as a technical one:

> My difficulty is not the general treatment of the case w^h seems sufficiently simple, but to suit my treatment to the circumstances as for example this that the Duke when he is ill does not think of eating or drinking less which you may believe would be the first thing I should be disposed to recommend to him. He eats a good dinner & takes just half a bottle of claret.[23]

By October Thomson had made some progress. His letters demonstrate that an intelligent practitioner could devise strategies to deal with even the most intractable aristocrat. As well as 'Keeping the stomachs of the various inmates in a proper state,' he reported, 'I have also some moral management to carry on.' The problem revolved around the Duke's own perception of his condition. He felt frequent pains in the back of his neck and attributed these to a cerebral congestion. Thomson was not inclined to argue with this diagnosis; but he did differ in the treatment to be administered. While the Duke demanded that he be bled, Thomson insisted on a more constitutional approach: he preferred purging to cupping.

It required considerable tact to ensure that his will prevailed. Thomson was solicitous about his patient's feelings and ever willing to concede that the principal goal of treatment must be to relieve these subjective symptoms. Thus, he 'begged [the Duke] at once to say whether there was any feeling of confusion in the head or other symptoms w^h appeared to himself to render it necessary to relieve cerebral congestion'. At the same time, however, Thomson gently resisted the Duke's wish for relief through cupping. He admitted to his father that he proceeded with no clear notion of the underlying cause of the symptom: 'Do you think it has its seat in the muscles or periosteum or in the upper part of the spinal cord?'[24]

He was, none the less, reluctant to acquiesce to the Duke's wishes, partly because bleeding appeared to depress the patient's spirits; but also because

> when he thinks he can have recourse to cupping he may eat and drink as much as he pleases. On this head I think he is gradually improving: he knows my sentiments upon abstinence very well, but avoids carefully any allusion to restrictions of this sort.[25]

In other words, behind the question of to bleed or not to bleed lay a struggle of wills between doctor and patient in which the latter pleaded for what he saw as a quick fix to his complaint while the latter insisted upon a thoroughgoing reform of the ducal lifestyle.

Thomson's difficulties in managing the Duke were, however, as nothing compared to the challenge posed by the Duchess of Bedford. She showed, he confided to his father, 'a certain want of restraint which at her age I should fear would increase'. Her heightened anxieties found expression in exaggerated concern for the health of the family:

> Thus one day when she is rather taking a gloomy view of things she will come to me & insist that 'the Duke is quite paralytic that Lady Georgina is as made of wax & that Lady Rachels bowels are overloaded to a great degree and the liver inactive.'

She was, moreover, Thomson told his sister, 'a great doctor and amazingly fidgety when any body is ill and fond of interfering with the practice'.[26] The Duchess insisted in short upon playing a traditional matriarchal role as the guardian of the health of her family – notwithstanding the presence of a professional male practitioner in the household. The Duchess's confidence in her medical skills rested upon the clear notions that she entertained of the workings of the body. When, for instance, her husband's stools were white she detected '"a total obstruction of the biliary passages" for which she considers calomel the only remedy'. She was no less certain about the state of her own health, maintaining that 'she is becoming dropsical at present and says she is breathless, which I think proceeds chiefly from the increasing unwealdiness of her body'. Dealing with all this eccentricity, Thomson wearily noted, 'requires some diplomacy on my part'.[27]

The Duchess, however, saw no need for such tact. Thomson complained to his mother that 'She seldom approves of my practice, always holding that two or three pills should have been given where I have administered one, and questioning the propriety of almost every prescription.' But such challenges to his competence were, in fact, salutary; Thomson claimed that he was now able to hold his own against his tormentor. Such confidence in prescribing was, he added, 'an essential requisite in a private practitioner'. The Duchess's revenge was to mock Thomson's prescriptions in public,

> particularly at the dinner table, 'There's a dish Doctor Thomson would recommend to your attention, it always requires to be followed by eight grains of calomel'. Then imitating my voice in the midst of the Dinner party she bawls out 'Your grace must excuse me I am determined to give no calomel'.[28]

Thomson was obliged to make his retort in private. He advised his father that 'I have examined the Dutchess' case & think obesity and flatulence the cause of her symptoms. What w^d^ you give to remove this!!!'[29]

During his stays with the Russells in the Scottish Highlands and in rural Ireland, Thomson was also introduced to a very different sort of medical practice. He 'neglected the sports of the field to assume the functions of a country Doctor'. In these remote locations he had to act as his own apothecary as well as physician and surgeon; but he was able to assure his mother 'that no lady has as yet had the indiscretion to ask me to fill the place of the fourth functionary of the medical department.'[30]

The patients Thomson saw in this capacity were at the opposite social pole to the Russells; they were among the poorest members of the population. They also belonged to a culture alien to a Lowland Scot. Because in the Highlands Gaelic was the prevalent tongue, he was 'obliged to have an interpreter for the greater part of my patients'.[31]

Thomson observed their ways with the same kind of scientific curiosity that Henry Brougham had displayed in his visit to the Western Isles (see chapter 1), tempered, perhaps, with a slightly more romantic sensibility. His practice had, he reported, provided him with

> considerable opportunities of seeing traits of the highland character and [I] should find it difficult to say whether the good or the bad predominates. It is in every way inferior to that of the lowland scot. Foolish family pride is the most prominent of the bad traits tho' not the worst. Cunning jealousy and servility are worse. On the other side of the picture we have devoted attachment which banished all selfishness and hospitality of the most open and frank kind.[32]

Like Brougham, Thomson found special interest in the economic conditions of the natives he studied. 'The farms', he noted, 'are small and even in the low land of the strath are chiefly for cattle'. The market had made little inroad; most of the grain produced was of coarse quality and was consumed locally. He was well aware of the link between the health and social conditions of his patients. Some of the chronic complaints with which he dealt were 'in great measure attributable to the poor living condition of the common people'. Their diet was, in particular, to blame:

> The fevers bear a typhoid character, most complaints are accompanied with considerable nervousness even hysterical symptoms, heart-burn is very common, and I think I am justified from these as well as other circumstances in supposing that oatmeal is not a wholesome article of food when not combined with something else[.][33]

Thomson extended his experience of the poor and their diseases while staying with the Russells in County Tyrone. He established a twice-weekly dispensary for the local population. Such an establishment was necessary because

> the poor people in the neighbourhood are miserably off for medical assistance, being attended chiefly by two or three old naval surgeons

> who are generally tipsy when they arrive at their patients & will not prescribe until they have received an additional supply of whisky.

So great was the demand for medical attention that Thomson found himself treating forty to fifty patients a day. As in the Highlands he was also obliged to be his own apothecary. He found such perforce 'hurried practice' most unsatisfactory.[34]

When visiting patients' houses Thomson again took on the role of ethnological observer. This might be seen as a perpetuation of the research strategy to which he had been introduced as a student member of the Plinian Society whose members' study 'besides the above mentioned objects [natural science] is directed towards the cultivation of Antiquities and the civil and natural history of Man'.[35] Tyrone, Thomson noted,

> is considered as the most comfortable & flourishing part of Ireland; They ought to have said the least wretched, – for throughout the district of 15 or 20 miles which I had an opportunity of observing, the instances of houses in which there is an approach to comfort are very rare indeed.

Nor was this impression the result of superficial observation: 'I was in the habit of going into all the houses & sitting on whatever I could find (a chair with a bottom being a rarity) entering into conversation with the inmates, learning their mode of subsistence their habits & wishes.' As in the Highlands, such living conditions took their toll on the health of the people: 'Pyrosis Dispepsia & Hypochondriasis in their worst forms and functional derangements of the heart occur to an enormous extent.'[36]

When confronted with similar poverty, the young Henry Brougham had blamed the system of land management. Thirty years later Allen Thomson preferred a different analysis of the roots of the problem. The land of Ireland was, he maintained, naturally fertile;

> The great want lies in the natural disposition & deeply rooted habits of the people. They are all careless & improvident in the extreme – even in the North where there is more similarity to the scotch and where in fact many families are of scotch extraction the people have the same fault and I think that in the most favorable circumstances the present and even a subsequent generation must pass away before there can be introduced those habits of steady industry & foresight which characterise the scotch peasant, with whom the Irish may be compared because he is not a bit poorer.[37]

In short, the poor were themselves to blame for their misery.

Thomson qualified this diagnosis to a degree. He recognized that the system of land tenure needed to be reformed before there was any real melioration. None the less, he placed far more emphasis upon the personal failings of the poor than upon the economic circumstances in which they found themselves. In this he was representative of the mainstream of contemporary Whig social analysis as expounded in the pages of the *Edinburgh Review* which saw coercing the poor to habits of industry as the only way to improve their condition.[38] Thomson approved the efforts of a local improving landlord to establish a factory on his estate, noting that 'labour is so cheap that one would think an establishment of the kind would be carried on with an easy profit'. He also maintained that 'the necessity of the poor laws for Ireland is pretty generally admitted by those who are not biased by party views and it is to be hoped that that part of the bill which provides for the employment of the able bodied destitute will occupy the greatest share of attention'.[39]

Despite these excursions into the Celtic fringe Thomson never lost sight of his principal concerns – medical politics and medical teaching. During a visit to London in the summer of 1836 he was able to expedite Sharpey's appointment to a chair in the University of London.[40] He also found time to conclude that 'there is no purer system of humbug than the greater part of London medical practice', and to treat the artist Edward Landseer for a head wound.[41] As part of the Russell circle he was also able to make many valuable political acquaintances during Whig social gatherings in London and at Woburn. In 1837, for instance, he was introduced to his grandfather's former lodger, Lord Melbourne, who, Thomson advised his mother, 'asked me particularly about you and all the other members of the Millar family'.[42]

Thomson was by now a strong party man who viewed individuals and institutions through Whig spectacles. These prejudices are evident in his account of the current state of the University of Oxford: 'You can have no idea', he declared,

> of the extent to which tory feeling and prejudices are carried in Oxford. The members of the University are exactly like the majority of the House of Lords and have not the slightest notion of what is going on in the world around them. They are all in a sort of politico-classical dream.

The reactionary nature of the university's politics had its effect on its academic vigour: Thomson noticed the tiny classes which scientific lecturers attracted in Oxford.[43]

Thomson did not lose sight of events in his own university. In October he discussed the future of the Edinburgh general pathology chair with his father and offered William advice on how to organize the course. Morbid anatomy, as it presents visible objects to the eyes of the pupils is undoubtedly the most attractive part and must for the present . . . take the most prominent place, but I hope that the great doctrines and more especially the Etiology will be discussed at length for this appears the most interesting to me and I know well that both the public and the students expect to have it. In it the most remains to be learned. And the cultivation of it will tend to correct the too prevalent error that General Pathology is nothing more than the study of morbid alterations of structure.[44]

Nor did his experience of medical practice – 'advantageous and improving' as it was – deflect him from his intention of following an academic career. He planned to return to Edinburgh in the autumn of 1837 to offer a course of anatomical lectures seeking to fill the gap left by Sharpey's departure. Thomson's bane, the Duchess of Bedford, intervened, however, to alter these plans. Their clinical disagreements notwithstanding, she was apparently distressed at the prospect of losing her resident physician and urged Thomson to stay. She had in fact shown some solicitude in attempting to meet Thomson's special needs when the family took up residence in Woburn Abbey. The apartment she chose for him 'is near a stair Doctor she said and you can carry any thing you are dissecting downstairs without going through the house. The windows open upon the ballustrade round the roof and you will be able to bleach your bones and skeletons nicely there.'[45]

Thomson was obliged to detail 'fully to her, the manner in which I had been occupied in Edinburgh, the circumstances in which I left it, and finally my reasons for returning, in respect of my desire to be established as a private teacher of Anatomy and my prospects at Glasgow'. The latter was a reference to the ambition that Thomson already entertained of succeeding James Jeffray as professor of anatomy in the University of Glasgow. The Duchess's response was to argue that, 'supposing the Glasgow professorship to fall vacant soon, that I should have a much better chance of success in remaining in the dukes family than in quitting it'. Aristocratic influence was, in short, allegedly of more moment in such matters than teaching experience.[46]

John Thomson urged his son to take John Allen's advice before making a decision. Allen, 'while he agreed with me that it was best for me to go home and be engaged in teaching Anatomy in case of any thing, yet he did not think that my *interest* would be in any way diminished (rather the contrary) by staying'.[47] What finally seems to have swayed Thomson was his father's opinion that

it will be necessary for you, in coming to Edin. to teach Anatomy, to bring along with you 2 or 3 hundred pounds worth of Anatomical Preparations and to have had an opportunity of practising Anatomy,

> and of Demonstrating all the parts and views Anatomical and Surgical, which may be required of you to do in the Dissecting room. He trusts that you will be able to carry on a good deal of this in London.[48]

In the event, the Duchess had her way; Thomson's return to the classrooms of Edinburgh was delayed until 1838.

Unkind cuts

Lady Holland is reputed to have introduced Allen Thomson to Lord Melbourne in 1833 as 'the future Professor of Anatomy in the University of Glasgow'.[49] The story may be apocryphal, but it is certain that no later than 1837 Thomson, urged on by his father, had his sights set firmly on the chair. The post had been held since 1790 by the septuagenarian James Jeffray (1759–1848); there seemed every reason therefore to hope for an early vacancy. With his Millar blood and political connections, Thomson had reason to be confident that he would be a natural successor. These aspirations were, however, for several years frustrated by the tenacity with which Jeffray clung to both life and office. William Sharpey expressed the frustration that this generated: 'I begin to think', he wrote, 'that old Jeffray's friends are using his name to draw his salary as some Chelsea pensioners have drawn their pensions long after they were dead & buried. Ought not a non efficient but salaried professor to be shown at stated times at Kirk or Market?'[50]

On the other hand, Jeffray's longevity gave Thomson ample time to enhance his qualifications as an anatomy teacher. He was, in effect, to take over Sharpey's class on his return to Edinburgh; and his former partner did his utmost to assist in this transition. In May 1837, for instance, Sharpey sent Thomson a suggested curriculum for a course of anatomical lectures.[51] He also offered advice on the accumulation of the preparations that John Thomson has regarded as a prerequisite for his son's course. In London, Sharpey declared,

> You can have what you like by paying for the *interment.* Sections of *heads, pelvises,* and their contents, ligaments &c. Prepared muscles &c. The only difficulty is the expense of spirits, but come yourself and then get down to Edinb. a considerable time before the winter, I regard that as of great consequence.[52]

After Thomson had commenced his course, Sharpey continued to provide guidance. On 24 November 1838 he congratulated him on attracting more than twenty students at his first attempt. Sharpey tactfully suggested, however, that Thomson's lecturing style '*wanted force*'. As for the practical aspect of the course:

> Let your manner be cheerful, good natured, never ironical, and in all important things serious and impressive. Don't get impatient with stupid lads, many a boy who annoys you by his apparent stupidity this year may delight you by his proficiency the next. Keep all the lounging and gossiping friends out of the Dissecting Room. And last of all dont be too anxious and distress yourself – *you are assured of success*, take care of your health.

As well as this general admonition and encouragment, Sharpey provided Thomson with a recipe for an antiseptic in which to preserve his subjects and specimens.[53]

Thomson needed all the counsel and assistance that he could elicit. It was, in the words of one biographer, 'no light undertaking at that time to become a teacher of Anatomy in Edinburgh'.[54] The memory of the Burke and Hare murders remained an irritant of deep-seated popular prejudices against dissection.[55] Despite the opprobrium heaped upon him in the aftermath of the scandal, Robert Knox remained an anatomy lecturer in Edinburgh. The Anatomy Act of 1832 was supposed to provide a legal source of cadavers: unclaimed bodies from workhouses and charitable institutions were to be made available to anatomists.[56] The application of this legislation in Edinburgh was, however, fraught with difficulties.

A letter signed 'Edinensis' to the *Lancet* in December 1838 placed the blame for early problems in the administration of the Act on David Craigie who was Inspector for Scotland. Since Craigie's resignation, the writer maintained, 'anatomy [in Edinburgh] has advanced much, and the supply of subjects has amply met the large demand'. As a result of these improvements, 'Our students now have every facility, not only of prosecuting their anatomical studies, but also of practically studying operative surgery, and at a cost very little higher than the vaunted economy of foreign schools'.[57]

This was an unashamed puff for the Edinburgh school; but even this optimistic author could not disguise that Craigie's departure had not solved all the problems with which the implementation of the Act was beset. Alexander Monro III, who had obstructed Craigie's attempts to control the supply of bodies,[58] continued to resist both the letter and the spirit of the legislation. 'Every unclaimed body', Edinensis complained, 'which dies in the Infirmary and is unopened, is sent, not to the teachers in turn, or in a ratio corresponding to the number of their students, but to the anatomical rooms of the University'. As a result, the university's dissecting rooms were filled with bodies 'from many of which no one ever derives any benefit'. Only 'mangled' bodies, unsuitable for dissection, found their way to the extramural teachers. Monro, in short, was seeking to exercise a monopoly over the supply of subjects in the city.[59]

This complaint was echoed in 1842 by William Campbell, director of the Edinburgh Funeratory, whom James Somerville, the new Inspector for Scotland,[60] had charged with ensuring an equitable distribution of bodies. In reply to a demand from Monro's assistant for a body from the funeratory, Campbell fulminated that

> Dr Monro has been in the practice lately of obtaining his supply from other sources without my knowledge and without any communication with or recognizing me on the matter, and certainly altogether exclusive of the arrangement alluded to by you, as made some years ago, with the sanction of the Authorities. That arrangement, Dr Monro certainly has *not* hitherto acted on, or adhered to; – and till now, never hinted to me his desire to carry it into effect. – In short, since I had charge of the Funeratory, he has stood aloof from its concerns and arrangements, – contributed next to nothing to its support, – Has taken his own separate and independent course, in procuring Bodies, – and altogether on his own responsibility, without my knowing any thing of the matter, except accidentally.[61]

A further difficulty arose from the reluctance of some of the municipal authorities to implement the requirements of the Anatomy Act. Of the three administrative districts of Edinburgh – the city, West Kirk and Canongate – only the first provided a regular supply of subjects for dissection. The other two, and the neighbouring town of Leith, provided only an occasional body.[62] The Royal College of Surgeons was obliged to write to the Chairman of the West Kirk Charity Workhouse urging him to co-operate with them to ensure the efficient execution of the Act.[63]

The response of the extramural teachers to these challenges to their livelihood was to set aside their normal habits of competition and to form an association to defend and promote their interests. Allen Thomson took a leading part in the work of this society. At a meeting held around 1832 a group of lecturers on anatomy and surgery committed themselves to a set of regulations drafted by William Sharpey intended to ensure the fair distribution of subjects for dissection. A rota was established to guarantee that, while the university professor had precedence, each lecturer would receive a supply of bodies proportional to the size of his class. The price of bodies was to be set at a meeting of lecturers at the commencement of each session; all cadavers were, moreover, to be procured through an officer appointed by the association and had to be accounted for by him. As well as this functionary, the society appointed a convener, a treasurer and a secretary. Monies for the purchase of bodies were to be collected from each lecturer.[64]

After Thomson's return to Edinburgh the lecturers were able to achieve a formal recognition of this arrangement. In Januaryuary 1840, thanks to the mediation of Lord Advocate Rutherfurd, an agreement regulating the supply of cadavers was drawn up between the lecturers and the university. Robert Christison acted as the university's representative at the negotiations; Monro was conspicuous by his absence. Under this treaty, all unclaimed bodies in the Royal Infirmary, the Charity Workhouse, or in the hands of the police were to be conveyed in the first instance to the Public Funeratory. There an official responsible only to the Inspector of Anatomy would take charge of the distribution of corpses according to a strict system of rotation.[65] It was Monro's flouting of this agreement that roused William Campbell's ire.[66]

The funeratory was seen as a key site within this system. It served as neutral ground where an impartial division of the spoils of the city's charitable institutions could occur. It was, moreover, considered less provocative to the public if bodies were routed through the funeratory rather than being transferred directly to dissecting rooms – 'a proceeding which from the habitual veneration paid by the people of Scotland to the Dead is attended with great odium and even with considerable danger'. Indeed, in a letter to the Home Secretary on behalf of the lecturers association, Thomson maintained that

> The greater facilities which the City has afforded for carrying the Anatomy Act into operation appeared . . . to have depended mainly on the establishment some years ago of a Dead House in connection with the City Charity Work House into which all bodies that are to be buried at the expense of the City must be conveyed; and from which such bodies as are not claimed are removed in terms of the Act to the Anatomical Rooms.

If the West Kirk, Canongate, and Leith parishes had similar discreet facilities, he argued, the supply of subjects from these sources would be greatly improved. He requested government funds for this purpose.[67]

Thomson was obliged to conform in his own practice to the regime that he had helped erect. When he complained in April 1842 about the state of one body allocated to him, he was curtly informed by Campbell that, according to the rules agreed by the lecturers' association, it was '*distinctly understood* that *no deduction shall be made on account of alleged mutilations*'. Should Thomson refuse the body offered to him at the set price, 'I am afraid it will count as one against you – or in other words you must wait [until] your turn comes again round.'[68]

Despite these difficulties, and in the face of stiff competition, Thomson was a resounding success as an extra-academical anatomy teacher. In the spring of 1839 only 18 students of practical anatomy were registered with him. Alexander Lizars, Robert Knox and Peter Handyside counted 125,

103 and 90 respectively. Within two years, however, Thomson had attracted a class of 65 for his lectures and 50 practical students. This placed him above both Knox (58 and 51) and Alexander Monro (50 and 28).[69]

The achievement is all the more remarkable because Thomson was not continually engaged in teaching in Edinburgh during this period. In 1839 he accepted the post of Professor of Anatomy at the Marischal College and University of Aberdeen. This may have seemed another step towards the Glasgow chair. Sharpey had in March 1839 advised Thomson of Jeffray's 'serious illness – from which it is said he will not recover';[70] once again, however, the old man was to confound these expectations. In the meantime a university appointment in Aberdeen would serve to bolster Thomson's qualifications when the happy day finally arrived.

At Aberdeen Thomson followed the same pedagogic strategy he had adopted in Edinburgh. There were, he advised his students, essentially two ways of teaching anatomy. The first was special or descriptive anatomy in which each texture and organ was described according to the system to which it belonged rather than according to its position in the body; thus the osseous system would be treated as a whole without reference to the peculiarities of the bones of any part. This, Thomson declared, was the approach best suited to beginners and the one he would adopt in his lectures. The second plan of anatomical instruction was

> that in which the student makes for himself an analysis of the structure of the dead body by dissection: by which means he not only makes himself accurately acquainted with the position, form, appearance & texture of the parts, but has also his Anatomical knowledge impressed upon his memory more firmly than can be done by any oral prelections.[71]

Because this form of anatomical instruction was especially directed towards the position and connection of parts, it was known as topographic anatomy.

While his morning course would be confined to descriptive anatomy, in the afternoon he proposed to give lectures and demonstrations designed to assist those more advanced students who were themselves engaged in dissection. Thomson pointed out that as most medical licensing bodies now required at least two courses of anatomy from candidates, it was 'desirable that all teachers of Anatomy, should adopt the plan of giving two different courses of lectures, the one elementary, the other more advanced'.[72]

Thomson provided a conventional rationale for the place of anatomy within the medical curriculum: its study formed 'in the practice of medicine the surest foundation for that scientific knowledge of the nature of disease which leads to rational plans for their alleviation or cure'. Just as in the

> mechanical arts the artificier must know the construction of the Machinery the motions of which he is appointed to regulate; so in the

> science [later amended to 'practice'] of medicine the physician and Surgeon ought to be familiar with the construction . . . of that most complex of all machines the human body.[73]

But he also went beyond such platitudes to emphasize the considerable variegation that anatomical science had undergone in the recent past. The subject had diversified in several branches each of which possessed its own rationale and interest. Two anatomical specialties with special reference to medical practice had emerged. The first of these was surgical anatomy: in addition to the knowledge of anatomy necessary to all members of the profession, the surgeon must

> possess such a minute & accurate acquaintance with the relative situation and appearance of all the parts, as to guide his knife with certainty in those instances in which it may be necessary to cut into the body, and in [the] greater number of instances to suggest to him other mechanical plans for the cure of diseases which it is the peculiar province of the Surgeon to superintend.

In the case of operations for aneurism, for example, it did not suffice for the surgeon to have a vague knowledge of the position of the artery to be tied;

> he must know perfectly all the other parts which are situated near the artery, he must even in some instances of extreme difficulty be able to recognize parts by the touch, and have that familiar acquaintance with them that an alteration of structure or position caused by disease may prove no hindrance to his progress.[74]

Such knowledge could come only through intensive and prolonged experience of dissection.

The alterations of structure and position caused by disease were the particular concern of another specialty: pathological anatomy. In late years, Thomson declared, this subject had 'received much attention and been greatly extended'. He forebore to mention the prominent role that his own family had played in this enterprise. He did not, however, neglect to assert the importance of these studies in a sound medical education. At the present time, pathological anatomy

> is . . . studied with assiduity by all those who are desirous of being distinguished as scientific medical practitioners; and will very probably soon be regarded in this country as it long has been on the Continent as one of the essential branches of study in a course of Medical instruction.[75]

Thomson also distinguished the general anatomy associated with the name of Xavier Bichat. This science showed that certain common textures were present throughout the organs of the body.[76] This study led naturally into 'minute' anatomy, a field in which 'the objects are frequently so small as to require the assistance of magnifying lenses or the microscope, – an instrument the uses of which in respect to Anatomy cannot be sufficiently extolled'. Thomson proposed to illustrate his teaching in this department with microscopic demonstrations.[77]

The enlightened anatomist, moreover,

> does not confine his researches to the structure of the human body alone, but draws from the Anatomy of animals illustrations of his own science. The study of the structure of animals, called Comparative Anatomy from the constant comparison which is made of with the well known standard of the human body, is not only one of the most interesting branches of natural knowledge in itself; but highly useful as affording a rich mine of extended illustration of the general laws of the animal economy which tend to throw light upon the human structure and functions.[78]

However, in Thomson's view, medical science had 'received a greater impulse and a greater addition of facts than from any other single source . . . [from] the study of the gradual formation of the young or the development of the foetus'.[79] Because embryology had revealed that animals of different classes developed according to the same laws,

> the study of the development in the primitive state comes to the aid of Comparative Anatomy in affording us a view of the simplest form of organs & structures so complicated in the adult condition of the body as to elude our search.

Related to the twin fields of comparative and developmental anatomy was 'philosophical' or 'transcendental' anatomy as propounded on the continent by Gustav Carus, Etienne Geoffroy Saint-Hilaire, and Johann Friedrich Meckel.[80]

Thomson ended his lecture by emphasizing that the study of anatomy 'does not belong to Medicine alone'; it was a legitimate area of study for all desirous of 'general information' about the sciences. This was especially the case when anatomy's relations to physiology were appreciated. Minute, comparative and developmental anatomy all involved the consideration of structure in its relations to function.

The scientific anatomist must perforce also be something of a physiologist: an 'intimate Connection' existed between these two branches of medical science '& diff[iculty]. of separating them in course of Lect. [is] at once obvious'.[81] This cognitive ambiguity could, however, also be a resource in shaping an academic career; it was to facilitate Thomson's next move.

The science of life

On 6 September 1841 Thomson advised Richard Owen that he was about to leave Aberdeen to resume anatomy teaching in Edinburgh. He had been induced to take this step

> partly from finding Aberdeen somewhat too much out of the current of science for my tastes and partly on account of my father who would otherwise from my brothers departure to Glasgow have been left quite alone.

There was, however, a further motive: 'reports are abroad that D[r] Jeffray intends resigning his Chair of Anatomy in Glasgow, and though I fear I may have but little influence I should like to take the field as a Candidate for the Office'.[82]

The main point of this letter was to ask Owen to amend a testimonial he had previously provided for Thomson. The alteration was small but significant; in place of the words 'Comparative Anatomy' Owen was to put 'Anatomy and Physiology'. Thomson was thus seeking an endorsement of his qualifications as 'a teacher and writer in Anatomy and Physiology'. This suggests that – Glasgow aside – Thomson had another possible opening in mind when he decided to return to Edinburgh; he had learned that the chair of the institutes of medicine would soon fall vacant.

In Augustust 1842 James Home, the Professor of the Practice of Medicine, informed Edinburgh Town Council of his resignation. The chair was promptly offered to William Pulteney Alison whose promotion meant that the professorship of the institutes of medicine was, in turn, available; Thomson made it known that he was a candidate.

The election to this post was contested. The Lord Provost put forward John Reid, who was professor of medicine at St Andrews University, for the chair. Thomson meanwhile was proposed by Councillor Macaulay. The issue was close: Reid received thirteen votes and Thomson sixteen. On 27 September a commission was duly issued appointing Allen Thomson as professor of the Institutes of Medicine in the University of Edinburgh.[83] He had thus succeeded where his father failed. At last a member of the Thomson family held one of the old chairs in the Faculty of Medicine.

The chair of the institutes of medicine had been established in 1726 at the inauguration of the medical faculty. By the end of the eighteenth century its remit was well defined: the professor was to teach the 'theory of medicine' comprising physiology, pathology and therapeutics. From the outset, however, Thomson made it clear that he had a narrower concept of the scope of his pedagogic responsibilities; in his first introductory lecture he insisted that he would confine himself to physiology alone.

This decision was, in part, an endorsement of the innovations that John Thomson had with such labour achieved in the medical curriculum. 'General Pathology', Thomson maintained, 'is now taught in the separate Chair instituted for the purpose'.[84] But he also maintained that the scope of physiological science was now such that a six-month course barely sufficed to do it justice.

Thomson thus placed himself in the tradition of Edinburgh teachers who had devoted courses to physiology alone. He was especially anxious to cite John Allen as a precursor. There were obvious personal reasons why he should wish to claim this lineage. When Allen left Edinburgh he had, moreover, bequeathed his teaching materials to the Thomsons; and these formed a resource that John and William later used in their own teaching. The younger Thomson in the course of his first physiology course similarly made reference to 'Allen's hypothesis of relative diminution of the power of the vessels [in inflammation]'.[85]

Thomson shared Allen's concept of physiology as a field autonomous of anatomy. His approach to the subject tended, however, to be more morphological than Allen's; 'The foundation of Physiology', he declared, 'is laid in Anatomy.'[86] General and minute anatomy were of particular relevance to an understanding of function. But Thomson did emphasize that 'There are limits . . . to the application of Anatomical knowledge to Physiological Science.' Certain functions, such as nutrition, 'are processes of the economy which cannot be explained by Anatomy'.[87]

Thomson's physiology moreover lacked the radical reductionist edge of his predecessor's. While John Allen was dismissive of all forms of vitalism and insistent on the application of physical laws to organic processes, Thomson adopted a far more equivocal stance. He was clear that for him 'life' was merely 'a general expression intended properly to denote the sum of a great number of phenomena'. It was, he added, an error to suppose 'the existence of an independent and separate principle an etherial something added to living bodies . . . through the agency of which all the Vital operations of whatever nature are carried on'.[88]

Thomson seemed also to echo John Allen when he maintained that

> The changes of the Nutritious fluid which moves through the body and the separation of the products of secretion are strictly chemical changes tho' they are not all analogous to the chemical changes which occur in inorganized, still a change in the elementary constitution of the substances takes place and this must be regarded as chemical in whatever situation or circumstances it occurs. [A]nd it is not unreasonable to suppose even that this chem[l] change is the result

> of chemical affinities [amended to 'laws'] such as we see acting in dead matter modified by some causes in living beings of the nature of which we are ignorant.[89]

The differences in the operation of chemical laws evident in the living body might therefore simply be the result of the different circumstances under which they there operated. But Thomson was far less categorical on this point than Allen had been; he presented it merely as a 'hypothesis'.

Furthermore, Thomson stressed that

> These remarks do not at all apply . . . to another class of vital phenomena which appear to be entirely beyond the reach of our investigations and of the cause of which we shall probably always remain ignorant. What prospect can we ever have to explain the operations of sensation judgement or Volition on chem[l] or mechanical principles. Is it not unreasonable to apply physical or reasoning on Material principles to that which is immaterial[?][90]

This was a far cry from the mechanistic theory of mind that John Allen had expounded in his dissertation before the Royal Society of Medicine (see chapter 2).

In the same address Allen had ridiculed the argument from design. Thomson, however, was willing to allow it. As a student in Edinburgh he had attended John Wilson's course on moral philosophy. He preserved his notes of the eighty-ninth lecture in which Wilson insisted that 'the belief of [God's] existence is produced and confirmed by the appearance of wisdom goodness and design in the universe'.[91] In his own teaching Thomson maintained that the support physiology gave to theism was one of its chief recommendations. 'Writers on Natural Religion', he maintained,

> in their search after proofs of the divine wisdom and goodness in the works of creation, have at all times drawn the greater number of their illustrations from the animal kingdom of nature; and justly so, for in the construction and functions of living bodies and especially of [the] human body, we meet at every step with the most striking and interesting examples of the unerring certainty of the operations of nature, and of beauty, harmony and design in the adaptation of means . . . to wise and beneficient ends.

Although he cautioned the student against confusing final with efficient causes, Thomson none the less insisted that

> the best arrangements of the facts of physiology are founded on the uses which each of the functions seems to serve in the great end of

> maintaining life, and that much of the interest which these facts possess depends upon one being permitted through them to trace some of the operations of the hand of infinite wisdom & power.[92]

Thomson was towing the party line. By the 1830s Henry Brougham, who at the turn of the century had sung the 'Marseillaise' and decried the twin vices of priestcraft and despotism, was a statesman who took time from his official duties to publish tracts demonstrating the value of natural religion. Central to the physiological aspect of this science was the doctrine that 'a given organ performs a given function . . . by its adaptation to mechanical laws . . . [And] that some power acquainted with and acting upon the knowledge of those laws, fashioned the organ with the intention of having the function performed'.[93] Thus,

> When we see that a certain effect, namely, distinct vision, is performed by an achromatic instrument, the eye, why do we infer that some one must have made it? Because we nowhere and at no time have had any experience of any one thing fashioning itself, and indeed cannot form to ourselves any distinct idea of what such a process as self-creation means.[94]

This form of physiology therefore insisted, not only upon the existence of the deity, but also upon his constant supervision and control of his creation. Another erstwhile Edinburgh Whig, Charles Bell, had with Brougham's encouragement given the fullest exposition of this form of reasoning in his treatise on *The Hand.* It must, Bell argued,

> now be apparent that nothing less than the Power, which originally created, is equal to the effecting of those changes on animals, which are to adapt them to their conditions . . . Neither can a property in the animal itself account for the changes which take place in the species. Every thing declares the species to have its origin in a distinct creation, not in a gradual variation from some original type[.][95]

These doctrines found exponents among extramural teachers in Edinburgh. In a popular physiology lecture given in 1836 John Fletcher (who had studied under Bell in London) declared that: 'It is on the evidences afforded by Physiology, of the wisdom, the power and the goodness of God, that the greatest men of every age have principally relied for inculcating a belief in the existence and attributes of a Deity'.[96] Fletcher made clear why it was thought important to insist upon these points; they served to refute the socially dangerous physiological doctrines promulgated by materialists. It was not, he maintained, 'among natural philosophers that we meet with the Tom Paines, the Carliles, the Hetheringtons, and the Taylors of this or any other age'. On the contrary, the 'pestilential precepts of infidelity have emanated . . . principally from benighted visionaries, alike blind to the beautiful harmony of nature. . . . A want of religion, revealed as well as natural, is not a mark of profound philosophy'.[97]

Despite his ritual obeisance to natural theology, teleology was not, however, the ruling concept of Thomson's physiological teaching. His leading idea was, instead, development. It was essential to grasp the historical dimension to organism: living beings 'pass through the stages or changes of growth of youth & maturity, when mature, produce others like themselves and then die'.[98] Because of this historicity it was possible to witness the gradual evolution of structure and function over the animal series as a whole as well as in the embryogeny of the individual.

This was a distinctly Germanic approach to the fundamental questions of physiology,[99] which Thomson had acquired in his student days. His MD thesis and early publications were essays in embryology.[100] In 1831 Thomson took part in a debate in the Plinian Society on Etienne Geoffroy Saint-Hilaire's views on the unity of organization. Four years later he delivered a paper in which he attempted to show the existence of creatures intermediate between the batrachia and fish: there were, he claimed, 'some genera of these reptiles which resemble the frog and newt in the tadpole condition, & which in fact might be regarded as tadpoles arrested in their development'.[101]

It was an orientation that Thomson retained to the end of his career. Speaking at the British Association for the Advancement of Science in 1871, Thomson sought to detach the notion of development from any specifically Darwinian connotation: 'the name of development is suggestive rather', he claimed, 'of that which seems to be the common history of all living beings; and it is not wonderful therefore that such a one should regard with approval the more extended view which supposes a process of development to belong to the whole of nature'.[102]

In its morphological aspect, this attempt to chronicle the process of development assumed the existence of certain organic 'prototypes' that were most clearly apparent in the structures of the lowest animals, but which were 'fundamentally identical with those of the highest'. Because of this unity of composition, 'the history of the advancement of each organ towards perfection is merely the history of the progressive development of an imaginary unity'. Fletcher noted that despite the strictures of Bell and other teleologists, such 'transcendental' doctrines were gaining ground in Britain – 'and even in Edinburgh a student does not *now* look quite aghast, as he was wont to do, when they are cautiously alluded to'.[103] In fact it was in Edinburgh that transcendental anatomy had boasted its most formidable British exponent. Since the 1820s Robert Knox had used the extramural school as a platform from which to criticize teleology and to expound more 'philosophical' doctrines.[104]

Knox's extreme political views served only to underline the dangerous character already ascribed to such concepts;[105] it was all too easy to see the law of the unity of composition as a confirmation of the physical descent of all organisms, including man, from some common ancestor. In his analysis of the theory of unity of type John Fletcher recognized this peril and argued strenuously against that system 'which would establish that "men and toads" differ only in their greater or less development'. Organisms were constructed, he insisted, not on one but on several plans.[106]

It was this attenuated version of the law of unity of type that Allen Thomson adopted in his teaching. His father had displayed a similar prudence a decade before when he succeeded in teaching Lamarckianism without evolution. Even in 1871 Allen Thomson was careful to distance the general concept of development from Darwin's version of the origin of species. When in a series of public lectures given in 1877 he at least hinted at his acquiescence in Darwinism, Sharpey reminded him that 'you dared not have said as much when you succeeded Alison in Edinburgh & if you had said as much before, the municipal Patrons . . . would never have promoted you!'[107]

To obviate these risks, in his Edinburgh courses Thomson concentrated on the unity of organization *within* the vertebrate sub-kingdom: he entertained no hypotheses about transitional types that connected vertebrate and invertebrate animals. It was, however, possible to see a gradual evolution of the major organic systems from a common type along the entire vertebrate series.[108] Thus 'A common plan of construction or type of conformation & structure of the Brain may be traced in all Vertebrated Animals from fishes to man.'[109]

This fact had important methodological implications. While many aspects of the process of human reproduction, for example, were inexplicable

> fortunately, the knowledge obtained from the observation in animals is very easily applicable to Man from the great general analogy w[h] is found to subsist in regard to some of the most important steps of the reproductive process, and in many instances where direct observation cannot be had recourse to in the human species the lacunae in the chain of facts are supplied from animals with almost equal certainty.[110]

In attempting to elucidate function the developmentalist strategy emphasized the need to identify the most essential forms of a vital operation in the lower reaches of the animal series or even among vegetables. Thus in his discussion of respiration Thomson noted that some animals breathed by means of lungs while others had gills. Some organisms, however, possessed neither of these mechanical contrivances: 'On this account I am disposed to regard the chem[l] part of the process the change of the blood as the most essential'.[111]

The task of the physiologist was then to chronicle the elaboration of this prototype to its fullest state of development found in man and other mammals. As in the case of structure, certain general principles were found to regulate the process of functional evolution. These rules of life were, for instance, evident in the case of respiration. Thomson maintained that

> In the lowest kinds of Animals this respiratory change is general over the body while as we rise in the animal scale we find that it becomes less so & a particular part is set aside for the function which is then more intimately connected with the Blood circulating through the Body.[112]

Physiological progress was therefore marked by an increased division of labour.

This metaphor had a few years earlier been made explicit by John Allen's former student Peter Roget who had argued that the organism could be compared to

> a chemical laboratory, where a variety of complex operations are going on at the same time. In the lowest orders of the animal creation, these functions are conducted in the simplest manner, and by the smallest number of organs. We may compare the reparatory system, in this case, to a manufactory on a frugal scale, conducted by ruder methods, with a scanty apparatus, and by the smallest possible number of workmen. In proportion as we ascend in the scale of animals, we find the processes extending in number and in refinement. The principle of the division of labour is introduced: the tasks before assigned to one and the same organ, being now apportioned among different sets of organs, the quality of the work is in the same proportion improved. In the higher classes of animals, the separation of offices becomes still more complete, and the products of one set of organs are passed on to the next in regular succession.[113]

The history of civil society and the evolution of the human body thus followed similar paths. Just as John Allen's notion of the self-regulatory properties of the organism referred to the hidden hand of the market, so Thomson's concept of development alluded to contemporary understandings of social progress. His was a Whig theory of bodily history.

Conclusion

In January 1848 Thomson finally received the news he had so long awaited: that of 'Old Jeffray's extinction'.[114] Sharpey encouraged him to exchange his present position for the vacant Glasgow chair. Apart from his longtime designs on the post, there were sound financial reasons for making the move. The institute's chair had never been one of the more lucrative posts in the Edinburgh medical faculty; and the 1840s was a period of falling student numbers. A professor like Thomson with no private practice and who did not exercise his right to take a share in the clinical teaching was especially vulnerable to such fluctuations. The anatomy class in Glasgow, although much wasted by Jeffray in his late years, was likely to provide a far more certain means of support.[115]

Although the structure of patronage was different, academic appointments in Glasgow were no less political affairs than in Edinburgh. The anatomy chair was in the gift of the crown although local interest could be exerted by means of the city's MPs. None the less, as Sharpey discerned, 'Lord John [Russell] and Rutherfurd ought and will . . . settle the affair.'[116] The decision rested, in other words, with two members of the Whig circle in Edinburgh with whom John Thomson had fraternized at the turn of the century. When his election was confirmed Allen was careful to remind Rutherfurd of this link between them: 'nothing', he wrote, 'concerning me could have given greater satisfaction to my father than my receiving this appointment, to which he from an early period encouraged me to look forward'.[117]

Thomson was to remain professor of anatomy in Glasgow until his retirement in 1877. As well as rebuilding the anatomy class, like his brother he sought to play the role of reformer within the medical faculty and the university more generally. Thomson also took an active role in medical politics at the national level; he joined the General Medical Council in 1859 soon after its establishment; and he took an active part in its efforts to renovate the system of medical education in Britain.

His departure for Glasgow marked, however, the end of the tale of the Thomson family in Edinburgh. The academic dynasty that John Thomson had strived to establish survived for only two generations. He did none the less leave a lasting mark on the Edinburgh medical school: although two of the Old Chairmaker's creations proved shortlived, the chair of general pathology endured. John Thomson's other legacy was the zeal with which his younger son pursued the interests of medical science in Glasgow while upholding the family's tradition of adherence to liberal principles.

Epilogue

In 1841 Professor K.F.H. Marx of Hanover made a tour of Scotland's medical schools. Edinburgh was his first stop. His visit encompassed the usual sights such as the museum of the Royal College of Surgeons and attendance upon such current medical lumiaries as Charles Bell and Robert Christison. But Marx also made 'a sort of pilgrimage' to Morland Cottage where John Thomson was living in retirement. Marx wished to make his acquaintance because 'for many years I had set a great value on the works of Dr John Thomson' and wished 'to know him personally and to express my gratitude for his important researches'. He was therefore disappointed to hear that Thomson had effectively withdrawn from Edinburgh society. With the help of William Thomson an interview was, however, arranged:

> We found the old man in bed; but I had scarcely had time to glance through the summer-house before he came to me, supported on a stick, and greeted me with affectionate cordiality. He took me by the hand, led me into the garden, thanked me for my visit. He spoke with so much animation, and such an unusual brilliancy appeared in his eye, and such tension in his sunken features, that I began to feel anxious for him and begged him to return. He seemed to suffer in his mind because many eminent men, with whom he was formerly on the best of terms, had criticised his scientific opinions in a harsh and unguarded manner. He mentioned particularly his views respecting the treatment of syphilis without mercury. He felt that he was misapprehended, and with this impression ceased to publish. . . . He leaves to his sons (the younger of whom, the professor of physiology, was present,) his valuable collections, that through these justice may be done to him.

There is a pathos about this account of John Thomson's last days. It shows him a virtual recluse shunning the medical society in which he had made his life. Although honoured by Marx, he felt he had little respect at home. After more than fifty years of unstinted effort to establish himself in Edinburgh medicine, Thomson remained an outsider.

This book began with the arrival in Edinburgh of two young men with a shared ambition to make a career in the medical world of that city. A central theme of what has followed has been the vicissitudes and contingenices that they encountered in the pursuit of that common goal. Some of the challenges that John Allen and John Thomson faced were common to any newcomer: they had to seek the competences, resources and patronage necessary to the creation of a successful medical persona. But their efforts were complicated by the fact that from the outset they identified themselves as members of the opposition to the prevailing system of power. Thomson and Allen sought an identity within the Edinburgh polity by means of antagonism as well as by identification. As a result their professional undertakings were imbued with political meanings; their career in medicine became the expression of a particular concept of citizenship. The fact that both chose to pursue a kind of medical career in which pedagogy played a central part ensured that this politicization of their professional activities would be overt and played out on a public stage.

Allen's case shows how medical discourse could serve as a means to demonstrate opposition to authority as well as to voice a critique of the cultural codes inscribed by that authority. This challenge to power was most overt, indeed blatant, in Allen's dissertation to his fellows in the Royal Medical Society. His later lectures on the animal oeconomy seem restrained by comparison; Allen the teacher skirted the delicate issues of mind and body that the student Allen had addressed directly. This course was none the less an event in the cultural politics of the city. It provided a opportunity for members of the Whig faction in Edinburgh to congregate and display their commitment to science. The concept of the living body that Allen expounded within this space was, moreover, one which was no less subversive for being more subtle than the doctrines he had enunciated on earlier occasions.

The wider significance of the utterances Allen made from an overtly medical platform were not lost upon those whom they were designed to outrage and unsettle. For his audacity he was effectively exiled from the city in which he had sought to make a life; and the subsequent attempt by his allies to rehabilitate him was firmly rebuffed. From his study in Holland House Allen might seek to pursue similar ends by different means. But the role of citizen-savant to which he had aspired was closed to him.

In contrast it was John Thomson's lot to endure to the end the trials of Edinburgh. He was a more subtle and pragmatic politician than Allen. He took care to avoid the censures of atheism and materialism that Allen had invited. Thomson did not seek to challenge his political enemies by the outspoken nature of his professed doctrines. His mere survival in Edinburgh was sufficient affront to them.

Without compromising his fundamental commitment to the Whig cause, Thomson was yet able to enlist the allies needed to achieve at least some of his aims. These allies included the officials of the army and navy medical boards, coloured illustrations of disease, and sundry Whig politicians. Most important among these allies were, however, Thomson's sons. William in particular was at first a mere appendage of his father, travelling afar while John Thomson remained at home or substituting in the lecture room when his father had to go abroad to visit patients. Eventually, however, William and later Allen Thomson were required to do more than merely serve their father; they were expected to perpetuate the ideals to which he had devoted his life.

Despite his early death, William gave ample evidence of both his capacity and his willingness to fulfil these requirements. But it was Allen Thomson who most fully enacted his father's designs. After 1848 Edinburgh ceased to be the scene of the Thomson family's attempts to combine the cultivation of medical science with the pursuit of civic virtue. The immediate scene of the endeavours shifted to Glasgow which in its academic polity presented to the Thomsons' eyes an egregious case of the survival of the old corruption. Allen Thomson's critique of these perceived abuses was couched in the language of Victorian liberalism; yet a residual debt to old Whig discourse remains. The familiar antithesis between vicious private interest and public virtue persists. But what is perhaps most striking about the terms of Allen Thomson's diagnosis of and prescription for the ills he observed in Glasgow was the prominence he gave to the ideal and practice of science as an instrument and object of reform. In the course of the first half of the nineteenth century the Philosophic Whig had undergone a subtle metamorphosis; he had become a liberal scientist.

Notes

Introduction

1. See Christopher Lawrence, 'Medicine as culture: Edinburgh and the Scottish Enlightenment', unpublished Ph.D. thesis, University of London, 1974.

2. [R. Mudie], *The Modern Athens: A Dissection and Demonstration of Men and Things in the Scotch Capital* (London, 1825), 221.

3. Christopher Lawrence, 'The Edinburgh medical school and the end of the "Old Thing" 1790–1830', *History of Universities* (1988), 259–60.

4. Michael Barfoot, 'Brunonianism under the bed: An alternative to university medicine in Edinburgh in the 1780s', *Medical History Supplement* No. 6 (1989), 22–45.

5. Lisa Rosner, *Medical Education in the Age of Improvement: Edinburgh Students and Apprentices 1760–1826* (Edinburgh, 1991).

6. Thomas Bender (ed.), *The University and the City from Medieval Origins to the Present* (New York, 1988), 6.

7. On the system of local government see T.C. Smout, *A History of the Scottish People 1560–1830* (London, 1969), 161–2; A.J. Youngson, *The Making of Classical Edinburgh 1750-1840* (Edinburgh, 1966), 46–8.

8. Mudie, *Modern Athens,* 182.

9. Anon., *An Examination of the Causes of the Declining Reputation of the Medical Faculty of the University of Edinburgh; and the Origin of Another Class of Medical Professors, Commonly Called "Private Lecturers"* (Edinburgh, 1834), 5.

10. Mudie, *Modern Athens,* 183.

11. Hugh Arnot, *The History of Edinburgh, from the Earliest Accounts to the Year MDCCLXXX,* 4th edn (Edinburgh, 1818), 405.

12. See Rosner, *Medical Education* (Edinburgh, 1991), 141–4.

13. See John Anderson, *A History of Edinburgh from the Earliest Period to the Completion of the Half Century 1850, with Brief Notices of Eminent or Remarkable Individuals* (Edinburgh, 1856), 279, 294.

14. Thomson's estate included £99 8s. arrears of his army salary: SRO, *Commissariot of Edinburgh,* vol. 69, pp. 774–5.

15. Margaret Thomson to William Thomson, 18 August 1822, NLS MS 9236 fo. 117.

16. Anand C. Chitnis, *The Scottish Enlightenment and Early Victorian English Society* (London, 1986).

17. Adrian Desmond, *The Politics of Evolution: Morphology, Medicine, and Reform in Radical London* (Chicago, 1989).

1 Philosophic Whiggism

1. H. Cockburn, *Memorials of his Time* (Edinburgh, 1856), 83.

2. For biographical information see P. Flynn, *Francis Jeffrey* (Newark, 1978); R. Stewart, *Henry Brougham 1778–1868: His Public Career* (London, 1985). On the ideas and significance of this group see J. Clive, *Scotch Reviewers: The Edinburgh Review, 1802–1815* (London, 1957); B. Fontana, *Rethinking the Politics of Commercial Society: The Edinburgh Review 1802–1832* (Cambridge, 1985).

3. Cockburn, *Memorials*, 85.

4. H. Cockburn, *Life of Lord Jeffrey: With a Selection from his Correspondence* (2 vols, Edinburgh, 1852), vol. 1, 66.

5. See Fontana, *Rethinking the Politics*, 6.

6. D. Stewart, *Elements of the Philosophy of the Human Mind* (3 vols, London and Edinburgh, 1792, 1814, 1827), vol. 1, 248.

7. L. Horner (ed.), *Memoirs and Correspondence of Francis Horner, M.P.* (2 vols, London, 1843), vol. 1, 104.

8. H. Brougham, *The Life and Times of Henry Lord Brougham* (3 vols, Edinburgh, 1871), vol. 1, 550–1.

9. The main source on Thomson's life is W. Thomson, 'Biographical notice of Dr Thomson', reproduced with amendments in J. Thomson, *An Account of the Life, Lectures, and Writings of William Cullen, M.D.* (2 vols, Edinburgh, 1859), vol. 1, 5–84. See also [W. Thomson], 'Notice of the leading events in the life of the late Dr John Thomson', (*Edinburgh Medical Surgical Journal* (1847), 131–93), which contains some details omitted from the later version.

10. Quoted in N. Murray, *The Scottish Hand Loom Weavers 1790–1850: A Social History* (Edinburgh, 1978), 161.

11. B. Thorpe, 'Biographical notices of the author', in J. Allen (ed.), *Inquiry into the Rise and Growth of the Royal Prerogative in England*, 2nd edn (London, 1849), xii.

12. Murray, *Scottish Hand Loom Weavers*, ch. 9.

13. Anon. to William Merry, 2 February 1817, BL Additional MS 48,431 fo. 51.

14. Thomson, 'Biographical notice', 6–8.

15. Quoted in W.C. Lehmann, *John Millar of Glasgow 1735–1801: His Life and Thought and his Contributions to Sociological Analysis* (Cambridge, 1960), 21.

16. Ibid., 26–7; Thorpe, 'Biographical notices', xiv.

17. Thorpe, 'Biographical notices', xii; Thomson, 'Biographical notice', 11.

18. On Allen's life see Thorpe, 'Biographical notices'; H. Brougham, *Historical Sketches of Statesmen who flourished in the Time of George III* (3rd series, London, 1843), 342–8.

19. Quoted in H.W. Meikle, *Scotland and the French Revolution* (Glasgow, 1912), 71. See also Thorpe, 'Biographical notices', xiii–xiv.

20. Ibid. 105–11. See chapter 2.

21. Thomson, 'Biographical notice', 14. A.F. Fourcroy, *Elements of Chemistry and Natural History. To which is prefixed, the Philosophy of Chemistry. With Notes, by John Thomson, Surgeon, Edinburgh*, 5th edn (3 vols, Edinburgh, 1800).

22. Fourcroy, *Elements*, vol. 3, i.

23. Thomson, 'Biographical notice', 14–15.

24. T.H. Shepherd, *Modern Athens! Displayed in a Series of Views: Or Edinburgh in the Nineteenth Century* (London, 1831), 63.

25. See Cockburn, *Life of Jeffrey*, vol. 1, 85–7.

26. [R. Mudie], *The Modern Athens: A Dissection and Demonstration of Men and Things in the Scotch Capital* (London, 1825), 187.

27. T.C. Smout, *A History of the Scottish People 1560–1830* (London, 1969), 373–4; N.T. Phillipson, 'Lawyers, landowners, and the civic leadership of post-Union Scotland', *Juridical Review* (1976), 97–120.

28. A. Murdoch, *'The People Above': Politics and Administration in Mid-Eighteenth-Century Scotland* (Edinburgh, 1980), ch. 1.

29. J. Clive, 'The social background of the Scottish renaissance', in N.T. Phillipson and R. Mitchison (eds), *Essays in Scottish History in the Eighteenth Century* (Edinburgh, 1970), 225–44. Cf. R.B. Sher, *Church and University in the Scottish Enlightenment: The Moderate Literati of Edinburgh* (Edinburgh, 1985), 315–16.

30. Cockburn, *Life of Jeffrey*, vol. 1, 84–5.

31. See S. Shapin, 'The audience for science in eighteenth century Edinburgh', *History of Science* (1974), 95–121; J.R.R. Christie, 'The rise and fall of Scottish science', in M. Crosland (ed.), *The Emergence of Science in Western Europe* (London, 1975), 111–26.

32. A.L. Donovan, *Philosophical Chemistry in the Scottish Enlightenment: The Doctrines and Discoveries of William Cullen and Joseph Black* (Edinburgh, 1975), 67–70; J. Golinski, *Science as Public Culture: Chemistry and Enlightenment in Britain, 1760–1820* (Cambridge, 1992), 31–2.

33. Cockburn, *Memorials*, 73–4.

34. Brougham, *Life and Times*, vol. 1, 87.

35. J. Dwyer, *Virtuous Discourse: Sensibility and Community in Late Eighteenth-Century Scotland* (Edinburgh, 1987), 190–1.

36. Cockburn, *Life of Jeffrey*, vol. 1, 54. Emphasis added.

37. Thorpe, 'Biographical notices', xv–xvi.

38. Sher, *Church and University*, 181; see also 187–90, 195, 198–9, 205.

39. J.G.A. Pocock, 'The varieties of Whiggism from exclusion to reform: A history of ideology and discourse', in his *Virtue, Commerce, and History: Essays on Political Thought and History, Chiefly in the Eighteenth Century* (Cambridge, 1985), 282.

40. See C. Robbins, *The Eighteenth-Century Commonwealthman: Studies in the Transmission, Development and Circumstance of English Liberal Thought from the Restoration of Charles II until the War with the Thirteen Colonies* (Cambridge, Mass., 1959); Pocock, 'The varieties of Whiggism'.

41. J. Brewer, *Party Ideology and Popular Politics at the Accession of George III* (Cambridge, 1981), part IV; H.T. Dickinson, *Liberty and Property: Political Ideology in Eighteenth-Century Britain* (London, 1979), chs 5 and 6; A. Goodwin, *The Friends of Liberty: The English Democratic Movement in the Age of the French Revolution* (London, 1979), ch. 2.

42. This paragraph is based on Robbins, *Eighteenth-Century Commonwealthman*, 7–11. See also Dickinson, *Liberty and Property*, 59–61.

43. Robbins, *Eighteenth-Century Commonwealthman*, ch. 6.

44. On the reform movement, see Meikle, *Scotland and the French Revolution*, chs 1–2.

45. A. Fletcher, *A Memoir concerning the Origin and Progress of the Reform proposed in the Internal Government of the Royal Burghs of Scotland* (Edinburgh, 1819), 182.

46. I. Hampsher-Monk, 'Civic humanism and parliamentary reform: the case of the Society of the Friends of the People', *Journal of British Studies* (1979), 70–89.

47. J.G.A. Pocock, *The Machiavellian Moment: Florentine Political Thought and the Atlantic Republican Tradition* (Princeton, 1975); 'Civic humanism and its role in Anglo-American thought', in *Politics, Language and Time: Essays on Political Thought and History* (London, 1972), 80–103.

48. Dwyer, *Virtuous Discourse*, 39-46; N. Phillipson, 'The Scottish Enlighten-

ment', in R. Porter and M. Teich (eds), *The Enlightenment in National Context* (Cambridge, 1981), 21–2.

49. Sher, *Church and University*, 191, 198, 205, 326–7.
50. Pocock, 'Civic humanism', 85, 90.
51. Pocock, *Machiavellian Moment*, 450, 466.
52. [J. Trenchard and T. Gordon], *Cato's Letters: Or, Essays on Liberty, Civil and Religious, and other Important Subjects* (4 vols, London, 1733), vol. 3, 27–8.
53. Pocock, *Machiavellian Moment*, 74.
54. On Fordyce see Robbins, *Eighteenth-Century Commonwealthman*, 211–12.
55. D. Fordyce, *Dialogues concerning Education*, 2nd edn (2 vols, Glasgow, 1768), vol. 1, 12.
56. Ibid., 13.
57. Ibid., 18.
58. Ibid., 24.
59. Ibid., 53–4.
60. Ibid., 33.
61. Ibid., 33–4,
62. Trenchard and Gordon, *Cato's Letters*, 31.
63. D. Hume, *Essays and Treatises on Several Subjects* (2 vols, Edinburgh, 1804), vol. 1, 119.
64. Ibid., 93–4.
65. J. Mackintosh, *Vindiciae Gallicae. Defence of the French Revolution and its English Admirers against the Accusations of the Rt. Hon. Edmund Burke* (London, 1791), 19.
66. Ibid., 328–9.
67. J. Millar, *An Historical View of the English Government, from the Settlement of the Saxons in Britain to the Revolution in 1688. To which are subjoined, some Dissertations connected with the History of the Government, from the Revolution to the present Time* (4 vols, London, 1812), vol. 4, 100.
68. Ibid., 168–9.
69. Ibid., 170–1.
70. Ibid., 304–5.
71. Ibid., 307–8.
72. Sher, *Church and University*, 10–11.
73. Cockburn, *Life of Jeffrey*, vol. 1, 94.
74. Cockburn, *Memorials*, 147.
75. John Leyden to Thomas Brown, 25 March 1798, NLS MS 3380, fo. 17. The full passage reads: 'So there is an end of my orthodoxy just when I had begun to be *flagrant* [sic] in the odour of sanctity and by dint of exclamation of every kind of French principles had become a general favourite with the *Terrorists* of Church & State. I do intend to describe by this term those who excite terror in others – but [a mistake for 'not'?] the Craftsmen who are terrified themselves'
76. Cockburn, *Memorials*, 148.
77. Pocock, 'Varieties of Whiggism', 308.
78. D. Forbes, '"Scientific" Whiggism: Adam Smith and John Millar', *Cambridge Journal* (1953–4), 643–70.
79. See S. Collini, D. Winch and J. Burrow, *That Noble Science of Politics: A Study in Nineteenth-Century History* (Cambridge, 1983), 44–5.
80. A similar engagement with different and in some respects contradictory discourses is apparent in John Millar's work. See M. Ignatieff, 'John Millar and individualism', in I. Hont and M. Ignatieff (eds), *Wealth and Virtue: The Shaping of the Scottish Enlightenment* (Cambridge, 1983), 341.
81. Horner, *Memoirs*, vol. 1, 79.

82. Francis Horner to James Reddie, 11 February 1806, NLS MS 3704, fo. 23.
83. Dickinson, *Liberty and Property*, 89.
84. Horner to John Archibald Murray, 24 November 1795, Horner Collection, LSE R(SR) 1054, vol. 1, fo. 3.
85. Francis Horner to John Horner, 2 September 1797, ibid., fo. 87.
86. Francis Horner to John Horner, 14 May 1804, ibid., vol. 2, fo. 105.
87. Francis Horner to Francis Jeffrey, 3 May 1805, ibid., fo. 197.
88. Brougham, writing more than thirty years after the event, was, however, able to take a more magnanimous view of Dundas: Brougham, *Historical Sketches* (1st series, London, 1839) 234–5.
89. J. Dwyer and A. Murdoch, 'Paradigms and politics: manners, morals and the rise of Henry Dundas, 1770–1784', in J. Dwyer, R.A. Mason and A. Murdoch (eds), *New Perspectives on the Politics and Culture of Early Modern Scotland* (Edinburgh, 1982), 210–48. For accounts of Dundas's life and career see C. Matheson, *The life of Henry Dundas First Viscount Melville 1742–1811* (London, 1795); H. Furber, *Henry Dundas First Viscount Melville 1742–1811: Political Manager of Scotland Statesman, Administrator of British India* (London, 1931).
90. Cockburn, *Life of Jeffrey*, vol. 1, 77, 78.
91. Cockburn, *Memorials*, 81.
92. Ibid., 87.
93. Ibid., 199–200.
94. Thomson, 'Biographical notice', 50.
95. Cockburn, *Memorials*, 283.
96. Thomson, 'Biographical notice', 50–1. J. Thomson, *Letter to the General Court of Contributors of the Royal Infirmary of Edinburgh; Containing Observations on the Minutes of Evidence, and on the Report of the Committee Appointed to Enquire into the State of that House* (Edinburgh, 1818); *A Second Letter to the General Court of Contributors of the Royal Infirmary of Edinburgh; Containing Remarks on the Proceedings at the Meeting Held on the 30th March, 1818* (Edinburgh, 1818).
97. See *The Scotsman*, no. 35, p. 279. The controversy over the management of the Royal Infirmary was, indeed, the occasion of the foundation of *The Scotsman*. See Magnus Magnusson, Matthew J. Moulton, William R. Monro, Philip A. Stalker, David Terris, Robert A. Warren and William Watson, *The Glorious Privilege: The History of 'The Scotsman'* (London, 1967), 3–4.
98. Anon. to W. Merry, 2 February 1817.
99. Cockburn, *Memorials*, 166–7.
100. Thorpe, 'Biographical notices', xvi. The passage continues: 'At this dinner a very amusing blunder was made by Mr S. of Culcreuch. . . . In the enthusiasm of giving a toast, he exclaimed, "May we all die like Hampden on the field, or Sydney on the scaffold."' John Hampden and Algernon Sidney were two of the martyrs of the Commonwealthmen.
101. Henry Brougham to Francis Horner, 5 September 1797, Horner Collection, LSE R(SR) 1054, fo. 89.
102. *History of the Speculative Society of Edinburgh from its Institution in M.DCC.LXIV* (Edinburgh, 1845), 378.
103. Ibid., 378, 380.
104. Ibid., 194, 380.
105. Ibid., 382, 381.
106. Ibid., 382, 28–9.
107. R.H.M. Atkinson and G.A. Jackson, *Brougham and his Early Friends: Letters to James Loch 1798–1809* (2 vols, London, 1908), vol. 1, 11.
108. ECA, Council Records, vol. 130, 1798–9, 375–80; quotation on 380.

109. Ibid., 383–4.
110. S. Shapin, 'Property, patronage, and the politics of science: the founding of the Royal Society of Edinburgh', *British Journal for the History of Science* (1974), 1–41.
111. Henry Brougham to James Reddie, 17 December 1796, NLS MS 3704, fo. 1.
112. John Rotheram (1750?–1804), Professor of Natural Philosophy. Rotheram had gained this appointment in 1795 through the influence of the Tory Hill faction in St Andrews: see J. Morrell, 'The Leslie affair: careers, kirk and politics in Edinburgh in 1805', *Scottish Historical Review* (1975), 69–70.
113. John Leyden to Thomas Brown, 14 November 1797, NLS MS 3380, fo. 11.
114. Leyden to Brown, December 1797, NLS., MS 3380, fo. 13.
115. John Hunter (1745–1837), Professor of Humanity.
116. Leyden to Brown, December 1797.
117. Leyden to Brown, 14 November 1797.
118. Leyden to Brown, 17 April 1798, NLS MS 3380, fo. 19.
119. Leyden to Brown, 17 April 1798.
120. John Leyden to Thomas Logan, 29 March 1798, NLS MS 3383, fo. 112.
121. Brougham to Reddie, 17 December 1796.
122. Henry Brougham to Francis Horner, 29 December 1796, Horner Collection, LSE R(SR) 1054, fo. 59.
123. See G.N. Cantor, 'The Academy of Physics at Edinburgh 1797–1800', *Social Studies of Science* (1975), 109–34.
124. Brougham to Reddie, 17 December 1796.
125. Cantor, 'Academy of Physics', 122
126. Fordyce, *Dialogues,* vol. 1, 58.
127. Ibid., 23.
128. Ibid., 66.
129. Ibid., vol. 2, 269.
130. Lauderdale to Holland, September 1798, BL Additional MS 51691, fo. 13.
131. James Maitland, eighth Earl of Lauderdale, *An Inquiry into the Nature and Origin of Public Welfare, and into the Means of its Increase* (Edinburgh, 1804). The book was very roughly handled by Brougham in the *Edinburgh Review*: see Fontana, *Rethinking the Politics,* 64.
132. See Cockburn, *Memorials,* 45.
133. Atkinson and Jackson, *Brougham,* 3.
134. Horner, *Memoirs,* vol. 1, 112.
135. Lord John Russell to John Allen, 30 September 1809, BL Additional MS 52193, fo. 167.
136. Lauderdale to John Allen, 26 November 1807, BL Additional MS 52180, fo. 104.
137. Lehmann, *John Millar,* 28, 38, 74.
138. [John Allen's political journal], BL Additional MS 52204A [27].
139. F. O'Gorman, *The Whig Party and the French Revolution* (London, 1967), 212–14.
140. Ibid., 166.
141. Henry Brougham to John Allen, [31] March 1800, BL Additional MS 52177, fo. 4.
142. Thorpe, 'Biographical notices', xvi.
143. Cockburn, *Memorials,* 147.
144. Cockburn, *Life of Jeffrey,* vol. 1, 85.
145. Cockburn, *Memorials,* 149.
146. Ibid., 148–9.

147. Brougham, *Life and Times*, vol. 1, 93.
148. Francis Horner to John Archibald Murray, 15 November 1804, Horner Collection, LSE R(SR) 1054, fo. 160.
149. Horner, *Memoirs*, vol. 1, 38.
150. Cockburn, *Memorials*, 187.
151. See J. Robertson, *The Scottish Enlightenment and the Militia Issue* (Edinburgh, 1985), ch. 2.
152. Ibid., 88–91.
153. See L.A. McKenzie, 'The French Revolution and English parliamentary reform: James Mackintosh and the *Vindiciae Gallicae*', *Eighteenth-Century Studies* (1981), 279.
154. Adam Smith, after extolling the martial virtues and comparing cowardice to 'leprosy or any other loathsome and offensive disease', went on to declare that: 'A man, without the proper use of the intellectual faculties of a man, is, if possible, more contemptible than even a coward, and seems mutilated and deformed in a still more essential part of the character of human nature.' (*An Inquiry into the Nature and Causes of the Wealth of Nations*, ed. R.H. Campbell and A.S. Skinner (2 vols, Oxford, 1976), vol. 2, 788).
155. Brougham to Robert Lundie, undated, NLS MS 1676, fo. 246.
156. Brougham, *Life and Times*, vol. 1, 106.
157. Ibid., 105.
158. See P. Wood, 'The natural history of man', *History of Science* (1990), 89–123.
159. Brougham, *Life and Times*, vol. 1, 106–7.
160. Brougham to Allen, 14 August 1799, BL Additional MS 52177, fo. 1.
161. Ibid.
162. Brougham to Allen, [17 August 1799], BL Additional MS 52177, fo. 3.
163. Brougham to Allen, 14 August 1799.
164. On the symbolism of the red cap see J. Harris, 'The red cap of liberty: a study of dress worn by French revolutionary partisans', *Eighteenth-Century Studies* (1981), 283–312.
165. Brougham to Allen, 17 August 1799.
166. Brougham to Allen, [31] March 1800.
167. Ibid.
168. Henry Brougham to Francis Horner, 6 Nov 1796, Horner Collection, LSE R(SR) 1054, fo. 51.
169. Ibid.
170. Ibid.
171. Millar, *An Historical View*, vol. 4, 142.
172. Ibid., 143.
173. Ibid., 144. Cf. Smith, *An Inquiry*, vol. 2, 784–5.
174. Ibid., 145–6.
175. Horner, *Memoirs*, vol. 1, 112.
176. Millar, *An Historical View*, vol. 4, 144.
177. Ibid., 146–7.
178. Pocock, *Machiavellian Moment*, 499.
179. Stewart, *Elements*, vol. 1, 224.
180. Ibid., 232.
181. See Fontana, *Rethinking the Politics*, 96. On the philosophical bias of Scottish education more generally see G. Davie, *The Democratic Intellect: Scotland and her Universities in the Nineteenth Century* (Edinburgh, 1961).
182. N.C. Smith (ed.), *The Letters of Sydney Smith* (2 vols, Oxford, 1953), vol. 1, 64.
183. Russell to Allen, 13 February 1810, BL Additional MS 52193, fo. 194.

184. Horner to Edward Adolphus Seymour, 11th Duke of Somerset, 14 February 1800, LSE R(SR) 1054, vol. 1, fo. 119. Cf. T. Brown, *Lectures on the Philosophy of the Human Mind* (4 vols, Edinburgh, 1820), vol. 1, 19–20.

185. Stewart, *Elements*, vol. 3, 259-60.

186. Ibid., vol. 1, 226–7.

187. Ibid., 228.

188. Ibid., vol. 3, 260.

189. Ibid., 332.

190. W. Erskine, 'Paper read before the Bombay Literary Society', NLS MS 3382, fo. 110, p. 120.

191. Leyden to Alexander Fraser Tytler, 12 June 1801, NLS MS 971, fo. 11.

192. Leyden to Thomas Logan, 21 January 1798, NLS MS 3383, fo. 109.

193. Stewart, *Elements*, vol. 1, 242.

194. Stewart, *Elements*, vol. 2, 439–446.

195. Cockburn, *Life of Jeffrey*, vol. 1, 103.

196. Horner, *Memoirs*, vol. 2, 392, 403–4.

197. Ibid., vol. 1, 49. Emphsis added.

198. Horner to Murray, 16 April 1802, LSE R(SR) 1054, vol. 1, fo. 154.

199. Horner, *Memoirs*, vol. 1, 51–2. 'Metaphysics and history, says Lord Bolingbroke in a very fine passage of his Letters, are the vantage grounds which a lawyer must seize, if he means to make a science of his profession' (ibid., 91).

200. Ibid., 55.

201. Ibid., 86.

202. Ibid., 78.

203. Ibid., 80–1.

204. Ibid., 84.

205. Ibid., 84–5.

206. Ibid., 111, 99. Italics in original.

207. For other examples see Brougham, *Life and Times*, vol. 1, 71; Cockburn, *Life of Jeffrey*, 103–4, 115.

208. Thomas Charles Hope to Robert Bow, 6 January 1800, ECA, College Miscellaneous Documents, Bundle 16.

209. [F. Jeffrey], 'Stewart's Philosophical essays', *Edinburgh Review* (1810), 168.

210. Horner, *Memoirs*, vol. 1, 182.

211. Horner advised his brother to attend lectures on political economy rather than chemistry in Edinburgh on the grounds that: 'Your Dr Hope is a sort of person that may be got at any time & at any place, if there is sufficient demand for such a commodity; but we are very fortunate if we have one Stewart in the course of a century' (Horner to Leonard Horner, LSE R(SR) 1054, vol. 2, fo. 52).

212. Quoted in Lehmann, *John Millar*, 83.

213. Thomas Brown held that there was a close analogy between the methods of the chemist and of the metaphysician: 'inquirer after inquirer, in the field of mind, may evolve to us unsuspected elements of thought and passion, as chemist after chemist, in the world of matter, presents to us elements that never had been perceived by us, in substances which may have been before us from the moment of our birth' (*Sketch of a System of the Philosophy of the Human Mind. Part First. Comprehending the Physiology of the Mind* (Edinburgh, 1820), 22).

214. Horner, *Memoirs*, vol. 1, 236–7.

215. Ibid., 111, 113.

216. Ibid., 237.

217. Horner to Somerset, 21 May 1802, LSE R(SR) 1054, vol. 1, fo. 160.

218. J. Black, *Lectures on the Elements of Chemistry, Delivered in the University of*

Edinburgh; . . . Now Published from his Manuscripts, by John Robison, LLD (2 vols, Edinburgh, 1803), vol. 1, 555–6.

219. See Golinski, *Science as Public Culture*, 148–50.

220. Horner to Somerset, 7 June 1802, LSE R(SR), vol. 1, fo. 170. Horner noted the anecdote that Lavoisier was led to see the necessity of a reformation of chemical terminology through reading Condillac.

221. Fordyce, *Dialogues*, vol. 1, 25.

222. Horner to Somerset, 17 June 1801, LSE R(SR) 1054, vol. 1, fo. 136.

223. Horner to Somerset, 15 September 1801, ibid., fo. 143.

224. Horner to Leonard Horner, 26 November 1803, ibid., vol. 2, fo. 56.

225. Cockburn, *Memorials*, 85–6.

226. Stewart, *Elements*, vol. 1, 269.

227. Brown, *Lectures*, vol. 4, 350.

2 John Allen, physiologist and Friend of the People

1. L. Mitchell, *Holland House* (London, 1980), 25. There are also a number of older histories of the Holland House circle: Lord Ilchester, *The Chronicles of Holland House, 1820–1900* (London, 1937); L. Sanders, *The Holland House Circle* (London, 1908).

2. B. Thorpe, 'Biographical notices of the author', in J. Allen (ed.), *Inquiry into the Rise and Growth of the Royal Prerogative in England*, 2nd edn (London, 1849), xix.

3. H. Cockburn, *Memorials of His Time* (Edinburgh, 1856), 177–8.

4. Ibid., 177.

5. Ibid., 80.

6. See H.T. Dickinson, *Liberty and Property: Political Ideology in Eighteenth-Century Britain* (London, 1977), 237–8; I. Hampsher-Monk, 'Civic humanism and parliamentary reform: the case of the Society of the Friends of the People', *Journal of British Studies* (1979), 70–89.

7. E. Royle and J. Walvin, *English Radicals and Reformers 1760–1848* (London, 1982), 64-5; A. Goodwin, *The Friends of Liberty: The English Democratic Movement in the Age of the French Revolution* (London, 1979), 283–4.

8. PRO HO 102/6, fo. 17.

9. Ibid., fo. 37.

10. Ibid., fo. 58.

11. PRO HO 102/5, fo. 373.

12. Ibid., fo. 318.

13. Ibid., fo. 369.

14. PRO HO 102/7, fo. 69.

15. H.W. Meikle, *Scotland and the French Revolution* (Glasgow, 1912), 71–2. In the government report on the gathering Allen is listed as attending with his uncle: PRO HO 102/4, fo. 344.

16. Thorpe, 'Biographical notices', xii.

17. W. Thomson, 'Biographical notice of Dr Thomson', reproduced with amendments in J. Thomson, *An Account of the Life, Lectures, and Writings of William Cullen, M.D.*, (2 vols, Edinburgh, 1859), vol. 1, 30.

18. Ibid.

19. Meikle, *Scotland and the French Revolution*, 256.

20. Ibid., 260. Meikle's transcription differs slightly from the spelling and punctuation of the original; I have used the manuscript version for this and the following quotation: PRO HO 102/6, fo. 383.

21. Ibid., 261.

22. PRO HO 102/6, fo. 381.

23. Goodwin, *Friends of Liberty*, 285–95.

24. 'Because we are friends of Reform,' Allen wrote in 1817, 'we lament the course lately pursued by Reformers. We can neither agree with them in their plans of Reform, nor applaud the measures they have taken for the attainment of their object.' In particular, he rejected the claim of these reformers that annual parliaments and universal suffrage were 'the antient and undoubted rights of the people' ('Annual parliaments and universal suffrage', *Edinburgh Review* (1817), 126).

25. Thomson, 'Biographical notice', 30.

26. Anon. to William Merry, 2 February 1817, BL Additional MS 48,431, fo. 50.

27. Thomson, 'Biographical notice', 31.

28. See J. Thomson, *Outlines of a Plan for the Regulation of the Surgical Department of the Royal Infirmary. Submitted to the Consideration of the MANAGERS of that Institution* (Edinburgh, 1800).

29. M. Barfoot, 'Pedagogy, practice and politics: The Edinburgh medical community in the 18th century', unpublished paper.

30. Cockburn, *Memorials*, 104–5.

31. [John Allen], *Illustrations of Mr Hume's Essay Concerning Liberty and Necessity; in Answer to Dr Gregory of Edinburgh, by a Necessitarian* (London, 1795). See M. Barfoot 'James Gregory (1753–1821) and Scottish scientific metaphysics, 1750–1800', unpublished Ph.D. thesis, University of Edinburgh, 1983, 300–5.

32. J. Gregory, *Additional Memorial to the Managers of the Royal Infirmary* (Edinburgh, 1803), 84.

33. Ibid., 92.

34. S. Shapin, 'Property, patronage, and the politics of science: The founding of the Royal Society of Edinburgh', *British Journal for the History of Science* (1974), 11–13.

35. Stewart forwarded a letter on Allen's behalf to the Home Office through the unlikely agency of Lord Castlereagh: PRO HO 102/19, fo. 55, 60. Lauderdale meanwhile solicited letters of recommendation from three other professors: Daniel Rutherford (botany), James Russell (clinical surgery) and Andrew Dalzel (Greek) (ffo. 57–8, 62, 66).

36. Francis Horner to James Loch, 5 January 1804, LSE R(SR) 1054, vol. 2, fo. 67.

37. For Addington's relations with Melville see H. Brougham, *Historical Sketches of Statesmen who Flourished in the Time of George III* (first series, London, 1839), 231–2.

38. Horner to John Thomson, 7 January 1804, LSE R(SR) 1054, fo. 70.

39. Horner to John Thomson, 10 January 1804, ibid., fo. 72. For the system of university patronage see chapter 3.

40. George Tierney (1761–1830) a vehement opponent of William Pitt and a maverick Whig; he was Treasurer of the Navy in Addington's government. Lauderdale approached Tierney on Allen's behalf (Horner to Loch, 5 January 1804) and Tierney wrote to the Home Secretary the following day in Allen's favour (PRO HO 102/19, fo. 64).

41. Horner to Thomson, 10 January 1804.

42. Henry Brougham to Horner, 10 January 1804, ibid., fo. 74.

43. See J.B. Morrell, 'Professors Robison and Playfair, and the *Theophobia Gallica*: natural philosophy, religion and politics, 1789–1815', *Notes and Records of the Royal Society of London* (1971), 46–7. Robison had asserted that 'the detestable doctrines of Illuminism' were being preached in Britain by such as Joseph Priestley. His strictures upon Priestley's theory of mind were equally applicable to the views expounded by Allen in his 1790 dissertation to the Royal Medical Society: *Proofs of a Conspiracy against all the Religions and Governments of Europe, Carried on in*

the Secret Meetings of Free Masons, Illuminati, and Reading Societies (London, 1797), 481–3.

44. ECA, Council Records, vol. 139, 14 September 1803 to 2 May 1804, pp. 220–1.

45. PRO HO 102/19, fo. 25.

46. Ibid., ffo. 30, 32, 34.

47. Ibid., fo. 47.

48. PRO HO 102/19, fo. 36.

49. Ibid., fo. 54. Horner had hinted that Addington might be deterred from doing anything to offend Melville whom he still hoped to win round to his cause: Horner to Thomson, 10 January 1804.

50. Ibid., fo. 23.

51. ECA, Council Records, vol. 139, 355.

52. On the Royal Medical Society see J.R.R. Christie, 'Edinburgh medicine in the eighteenth century; the view from the students', *Bulletin of the Society for the Social History of Medicine* (1976), 13–15; Christopher Lawrence, 'Medicine as culture: Edinburgh and the Scottish Enlightenment', unpublished Ph.D. thesis, University of London 1984, 200–17; L. Rosner, *Medical Education in the Age of Improvement: Edinburgh Students and Apprentices 1760–1826* (Edinburgh, 1991), 119–34.

53. J. Mackintosh, *Memoirs of the Life of the Right Honourable Sir James Mackintosh*, 2nd edn (2 vols, London, 1836), vol. 1, 26.

54. James Gregory, *Memorial to the managers of the Royal Infirmary. MDCCC*, 2nd edn (Edinburgh, 1803), 395.

55. Ibid., 384–5.

56. M. Barfoot, 'Brunonianism under the bed: an alternative to university medicine in Edinburgh in the 1780s', *Medical History*, Supplement No. 8 (1988), 42.

57. *Caledonian Mercury*, 10 March 1792. Quoted in Meikle, *Scotland and the French Revolution*, 78.

58. The continuity with the era of the Brunonian debates may have been still stronger. A. Philips Wilson recalled that 'in the Medical Society of Edinburgh I have often heard Mr Allen, with much perspicuity, defend his opinion of the proximate causes of inflammation'. This theory was Brunonian inasmuch as it attributed inflammation to a debility of the blood vessels (*A Treatise on Febrile Diseases, including Intermitting, Remitting, and Continued Fevers; Eruptive Fevers; Inflammations; Hemorrhagies; and the Profluvia* (4 vols, Winchester, 1801), vol. 3, 25–6). During the 1795–6 session, Allen continued to maintain that 'in cases of gen[l] inflam[n] attended with phlogistic or sthenic diathesis, y[e] action of the vessels is said to be less than those of the system in general' (W. Henry, 'Lectures on the animal oeconomy by Mr John Allen. Edinburgh – 1795,6', John Rylands Library Manchester, AN.A91, 33–4).

59. RMS List of Dissertations, vol. 25, 41–65.

60. J. Allen, ['Mania'], GUL MS Gen. 1476, Box 26, 1.

61. Ibid., 2–3.

62. Ibid., 3–4.

63. Ibid., 10–11.

64. Ibid., 11. This is a close paraphrase of Hume's own words: 'An inquiry concerning human understanding', *Essays and Treatises on Several Subjects* (2 vols, Edinburgh, 1804), vol. 2, 23-4.

65. Ibid., 13–14.

66. Ibid., 17.

67. Ibid., 19.

68. Ibid., 19–21.

69. Ibid., 21.

70. Ibid., 22.

71. D. Stewart, *Outlines of Moral Philosophy: For the Use of Students in the University of Edinburgh* (Edinburgh, 1793), 148–9.

72. Ibid., 150.

73. D. Stewart, *Philosophical Essays* (Edinburgh, 1810), 127; *Elements of the Philosophy of the Human Mind* (3 vols, London and Edinburgh, 1792, 1814, 1827), vol. 2, 425–6.

74. Allen, however, maintained that a theory that saw the mind purely as an aggregate of sensations 'differs from every system which asserts either the *materiality* or *immateriality* of the Soul. It is in direct contradiction to both alleging only that certain changes in the Brain are followed by certain Sensations, but denying that these sensations have any substance or connecting Medium, either material, or spiritual.' This he regarded as Hume's position. ([Notes on physiology], BL Additional MS 52245, pp. 88–9).

75. Francis Horner recalled that Lady Blair used to say of Allen that he was 'not only a Deist but an Atheist' (Horner to Dugald Stewart, 12 February 1806, LSE R(SR), vol. 2, fo. 21).

76. D. Stewart, *The Philosophy of the Active and Moral Powers of Man* (2 vols, Edinburgh, 1828), vol. 1, vi.

77. Allen's class lists are in GUL MS Gen. 1476, Box 18. Allen's auditors included: John Barclay (1796); Charles Bell (1795); George Birkbeck (1797, 1798); John Bostock (1796); Thomas Brown (1799, 1802); John Gordon (1802); Francis Horner (1799); Robert Jameson (1794, 1795, 1796); John Leyden (1798); Peter Roget (1795, 1796, 1797); and John Thomson (1794, 1795).

78. 'Lectures on the animal oeconomy', BL Additional MS 5221, 5.

79. Henry, 'Lectures', 273–83.

80. A.R. Cunningham, 'Aspects of the history of medical education in Britain in the 17th and early 18th centuries', unpublished Ph.D. thesis, University of London, 1974, 134–9; Lawrence, 'Medicine as culture', 39–48, 146–7, 322–3.

81. H.C. Boisragon, '1797. Lectures on the animal oeconomy, by Mr John Allen', 3 vols, EUL MS Gen. 2007/6, vol. 3, 45.

82. Henry, 'Lectures', 196.

83. Ibid., 240.

84. Boisragon, 'Lectures', vol. 1, 170.

85. Ibid., 65–7.

86. Ibid., 81.

87. Allen, 'Lectures on the animal oeconomy' (British Library).

88. Ibid.

89. Henry, 'Lectures', 1.

90. Christopher Lawrence, 'The nervous system and society in the Scottish Enlightenment', in B. Barnes and S. Shapin (eds), *Natural Order: Historical Studies of Scientific Culture* (Beverly Hills and London,), 19. See also: idem, 'Medicine as culture', 428–9.

91. H. Brougham, *Historical Sketches* (3rd series, London, 1843) 343.

92. See the unfavourable comments on Bonaparte's government in Allen to Francis Horner, 18 August 1802, LSE R(SR), vol. 1, fo. 180. Allen recognized Napoleon's many personal qualities; ultimately, however, he failed the civic humanist test of virtue: '[Napoleon's] views were all personal and selfish. . . . He might have established a republick: To found a dynasty of Kings was his ambition' ('Napoleon Bonaparte', *Edinburgh Review* (1816), 480).

93. Allen to Macvey Napier, [9 August 1830], BL Additional MS 34 614, fo. 369.

94. Boisragon, 'Lectures', vol. 1, 69.
95. Ibid., vol. 2, 83.
96. Golinski has shown how Edmund Burke employed chemical metaphors in his castigation of the mentality that had led to the Revolution in France: J. Golinski, *Science as Public Culture, Chemistry and Enlightenment in Britain, 1760–1820* (Cambridge, 1992), 176–7.
97. J. Black, *Lectures on the Elements of Chemistry, Delivered in the University of Edinburgh; . . . Now Published from his Manuscripts, by John Robison, LLD.* (2 vols, Edinburgh, 1803), vol. 1, 555–6. See Morrell, 'Professors Robison and Playfair', 50–1; A. Donovan, 'Scottish responses to the new chemistry of Lavoisier', *Studies in Eighteenth-Century Culture* (1979), 246–7.
98. Boisragon, 'Lectures', vol. 1, 160.
99. Henry, 'Lectures', 13.
100. Boisragon, 'Lectures', vol. 1, 9.
101. Ibid., 160–2.
102. Ibid., 162. J.J. Plenck, *The Hygrology, or Chemico-Physiological Doctrine of the Fluids of the Human Body* (London, 1797), 256–7.
103. Boisragon, 'Lectures', vol. 2, 55–7. G. Fordyce, *A Treatise on the Digestion of Food* (London, 1791), 171–2.
104. Boisragon, 'Lectures', 25–7, 29.
105. Ibid., vol. 1, 72.
106. Ibid., 107–8.
107. Henry, 'Lectures', 36.
108. Ibid., 38.
109. Thomas Thomson, *A System of Chemistry* (4 vols, Edinburgh, 1802), vol. 4, 519–20.
110. Ibid., 523.
111. L.S. Jacyna, 'Immanence or transcendence: theories of life and organization in Britain, 1790–1835', *Isis* (1983), 85–108. Thomson's views were reproduced in one of the most important texts of these controversies: John Barclay, *An Inquiry into the Opinions, Ancient and Modern, Concerning Life and Organization* (Edinburgh, 1822), 390–2. Barclay had attended Allen's lectures in 1796.
112. J. Barclay, 'Physiology', *Encyclopaedia Britannica*, 3rd edn (Edinburgh, 1797), 667, 668. Barclay's political orientation can be inferred from his association with the rabidly Tory *Anti-Jacobin Review* in which he published a number of articles. See E.L. de Montluzin, *The Anti-Jacobins 1798–1800: The Early Contributors to the Anti-Jacobin Review*, (London, 1988), 56–7.
113. See A. Smith, *An Inquiry into the Nature and Causes of the Wealth of Nations*, ed. R.H. Campbell and A.S. Skinner (2 vols, Oxford, 1976), vol. 2, 687. In Dugald Stewart's view, 'the great and leading object of [Smith's] speculations' was to demonstrate that 'the most effectual plan for advancing a people to greatness, is to maintain that order of things which nature has pointed out, by allowing every man . . . to pursue his own interest in his own way, and to bring both his industry and his capital into the freest competition with those of his fellow-citizens' ('Account of the life and writings of Adam Smith LL.D', in *The Collected Works of Dugald Stewart*, ed. W. Hamilton (10 vols, Edinburgh, 1858), vol. 10, 60).
114. Stewart, *Elements*, vol. 1, 242.
115. Thomson, *System of Chemistry*, vol. 4, 520–1.
116. For a similar interpretation of John Hunter's physiology see S.J. Cross, 'John Hunter, the animal oeconomy, and late eighteenth-century physiological discourse', *Studies in History of Biology* (1981), 74–5. In flights of poetic fancy, eighteenth-century authors sometimes made the parallels between body and state explicit:

How utter by what exquisite design
The *nervous* substance, in connected chain,
Runs through the long articulated Spine!
. . .
So through the Nerves the Spirits, from each part,
Winged Intelligencers, bear at once
Their Information to the *imperial* Brain;
Who, as true sovereign of the commonwealth,
Feels *all* their Good, and suffers *all* their Ill.

(C. Lofft, *Eudosia: Or, a Poem on the Universe* (London, 1781), 158, 171.)

117. Henry, 'Lectures', 218–21.
118. Boisragon, 'Lectures', vol. 3, 110.
119. Ibid., 161.
120. Ibid., 157–9.
121. On these controversies see S.A. Roe, 'Rationalism and embryology: Caspar Friedrich Wolff's theory of epigenesis', *Journal of the History of Biology* (1979), 1–43; *Matter, Life, and Generation: Eighteenth-Century Embryology and the Haller-Wolff Debate* (Cambridge, 1981); 'Voltaire *vs.* Needham: atheism, materialism, and the generation of life', *Journal of the History of Ideas* (1985), 65–87.
122. J. Allen, *An Introduction to the Study of the Animal Economy; Translated from the French of Cuvier, by John Allen, Fellow of the Royal College of Surgeons, and Lecturer on the Animal Economy, at Edinburgh* (Edinburgh, 1801), [ii].
123. Ibid., 1.
124. Ibid., 5.
125. Ibid., 6.
126. G.L. Geison, *Michael Foster and the Cambridge School of Physiology: The Scientific Enterprise in Late Victorian Society* (Princeton, 1978), 18–31.
127. Barclay, 'Physiology', 668–9. Allen's reading of Cuvier was, of course, highly selective; the latter's methodological pronouncements stressed the intimacy between anatomical and physiological knowledge.
128. L. Horner (ed.), *Memoirs and Correspondence of Francis Horner, M.P.* (2 vols, London, 1843), vol. 1, 89.
129. C. Standish to John Allen, [January 1815], BL Additional MS 52194 fo. 72; Allen to Standish, January 1815, fo. 74.
130. Leonard Horner to Allen, 27 September 1816, ibid., fo. 74; see also fo. 87.
131. John Thomson to Allen, 4 October 1819, ibid., fo. 131. Allen's record of the case is in BL Additional MS 52,208.
132. Matthew Baillie to Allen, 2 November 1819, ibid., fo. 143.
133. John William Turner to Allen, 28 April 1830, BL Additional MS 52196, fo. 42.
134. [J. Allen], *Thoughts on Medical Reform. By a Retired Practitioner* (London, 1833), 3.
135. Ibid., 16, 28.
136. Charles Bell to Allen, 11 December 1811, BL Additional MS 52194, fo. 12.
137. See E. Clarke and L.S. Jacyna, *Nineteenth-Century Origins of Neuroscientific Concepts* (Berkeley, 1987), 110–11. Bell also sought Allen's advice in 1835 on the advisability of returning to Edinburgh to take up the chair of surgery. Bell to Allen, 1 December [1835], BL Additional MS 52197, fo. 20.
138. Dugald Stewart to Allen, 2 February 1813, BL Additional MS 52194, fo. 48.
139. See J.G.A. Pocock, 'The varieties of Whiggism from exclusion to reform: a history of ideology and discourse', in *Virtue, Commerce, and History: Essays on Political Thought and History in the Eighteenth Century* (Cambridge, 1985), 300.

140. Brougham's review is reproduced in Allen, *Inquiry*, xxxi.
141. Ibid., xxxii–xxxiii.
142. J. Allen (ed.), *Inquiry into the Rise and Growth of the Royal Prerogative in England* (London, 1830), 2.
143. Ibid., 164.
144. Ibid., 2.
145. Allen to Macvey Napier, 6 June 1837, BL Additional MS 34618, fo. 148.
146. Allen, *Inquiry* (1830), 51.
147. Ibid., 27–8. See E.H. Kantorowicz, *The King's Two Bodies: A Study in Medieval Political Theology* (Princeton, 1961).
148. Ibid., 29.
149. J. Allen, *Vindication of the Ancient Independence of Scotland* (London, 1833), 3–4.
150. See J.G.A. Pocock, *The Machiavellian Moment: Florentine Political Thought and the Atlantic Republican Tradition* (Princeton, 1975), 476; M.C. Jacob, *The Radical Enlightenment: Pantheists, Freemasons and Republicans* (London, 1981), 149–50 and *passim*.

3 The Old Chairmaker

1. 'Bruinowsky', *An Answer to the Verses, Lately Published by William Smith in Regard to the Raising of the Dead; with some Reflections suggested thereby* (Edinburgh, 1820?), 7.
2. *Lancet* (1833–4) 1, 730.
3. The exception was the chair of botany where there was an obscure and contentious dual patronage by the Town Council and crown.
4. On the history of the university see A. Grant, *The Story of the University of Edinburgh during its First Three Hundred Years* (2 vols, Edinburgh, 1884); D.B. Horn, *A Short History of the University of Edinburgh 1556–1889* (Edinburgh, 1967).
5. See L.J. Saunders, *Scottish Democracy 1815–1840: The Social and Intellectual Background* (Edinburgh, 1950), 315–16.
6. H. Arnot, *The History of Edinburgh, From the Earliest Accounts to the Year MDCCLXXX*, 4th edn (Edinburgh, 1818), 392.
7. A.J. Youngson, *The Making of Classical Edinburgh 1750–1840* (Edinburgh, 1966), 47.
8. J.B. Morrell, 'The Edinburgh Town Council and its university, 1717–1766', in R.G.W. Anderson and A.D.C. Simpson (eds), *The Early Years of the Edinburgh Medical School* (Edinburgh, 1976).
9. [R. Mudie], *The Modern Athens: A Dissection and Demonstration of Men and Things in the Scotch Capital* (London, 1825), 212.
10. Ibid., 213.
11. H. Monteith to Robert Saunders Dundas, second Viscount Melville, 18 December 1819, WIHM MS 5122, 1–31.
12. Letter of 24 October 1798, ECA, College Miscellaneous Documents, Bundle 16. The memorial was in response to an attempt to create a chair of medical jurisprudence in the university.
13. J.B. Morrell, 'The University of Edinburgh: its scientific eminence and academic structure', *Isis* (1970), 160–1.
14. Grant, *Story of the University of Edinburgh*, 290–2.
15. 'Report relative to the new chair in the University 6 December 1816', ECA College Miscellaneous Documents, Bundle 16, pp. 9–10.
16. Ibid., 9.

17. Ibid., 6.

18. 'Report of the committee appointed by the Senatus Academicus to consider the Communication by the Right Hon[ble] The Lord Provost, relative to the appointment of a Professorship of Comparative Anatomy and of Veterinary Physic and Surgery', ECA College Miscellaneous Documents, Bundle 16.

19. Alexander Monro to William Arbuthnot, 3 September 1816, ibid.

20. See R.M. Sunter, *Patronage and Politics in Scotland, 1707–1832* (Edinburgh, 1986), 28–9, 72–3.

21. Henry Richard Lord Holland, *Memoirs of the Whig Party during my Time* (2 vols, London, 1852), vol. 1, 243.

22. George H. Baird to Melville, 8 August 1821, WIHM MS 5122/32–63.

23. James Finlayson to Robert Dundas, 1 April 1801, ibid., 5120/39–57. Finlayson was later to play the leading role in the attempt to exclude John Leslie from the professoriate because of his alleged religious heterodoxy.

24. F. Horner to F. Jeffrey, 13 June 1806, LSE MS R(SR) 1054, vol. 3, fo. 64.

25. 'Case of the lectureship of the Materia Medica in the University of Glasgow', SRO HH5/6.

26. John Douglas to Melbourne, 26 January 1831, SRO HH5/6.

27. Jeffrey to Melbourne, 15 July 1831, SRO HH5/6.

28. J. Millar, *An Historical View of the English Government, from the Settlement of the Saxons in Britain to the Revolution of 1688. To which are subjoined, some Dissertations connected with the History of the Government, from the Revolution to the Present Time* (4 vols, London, 1812), vol. 4, 95–7.

29. Jeffrey to Allen, 17 March 1807, BL Additional MS 52181, fo. 2.

30. On medical education in Edinburgh see L. Rosner, *Medical Education in the Age of Improvement: Edinburgh Students and Apprentices 1760–1826* (Edinburgh, 1991).

31. Ibid., 86–103, 141–60.

32. Christopher Lawrence, 'The Edinburgh medical school and the end of the "Old Thing" 1790–1830', *History of Universities* (1988), especially 263.

33. GUL MS Gen. 1476, Box 2.

34. Rosner, *Medical Education*, 149.

35. J. Russell, 'Memorial in favour of the erection of a clinical & pathological professor of surgery in the university of Edinburgh', EUL MS, La II 500, p. 8.

36. Ibid. 9. Russell was also careful to make the point that his father had been a professor in the university.

37. There is no satisfactory study of the impact of war on medicine at the turn of the nineteenth century; but see Peter Mathias, 'Swords and ploughshares: the armed forces, medicine and public health in the late eighteenth century', in J.M. Winter (ed.), *War and Economic Development* (Cambridge, 1975), 73–90.

38. Especially after the appointment of James M[c]Grigor to the Army Medical Board in 1815 there was a deliberate attempt to improve the education of medical officers and to link promotion to academic qualifications. See J. M[c]Grigor, *The Autobiography and Services of Sir James M[c]Grigor, Bart.* (London, 1861), 95–6. The policy was formalized in a memorandum of 1826: PRO WO 30/139, fo. 228.

39. W. Thomson, 'Biographical notice of Dr Thomson', reproduced with amendments in J. Thomson, *An Account of the Life, Lectures, and Writings of William Cullen, M.D.* (2 vols, Edinburgh, 1859), vol. 1, 12–13.

40. See E.W. Wall, 'John Bell, 1763–1820', *Medical History* (1964), 63–9.

41. Thomson, 'Biographical notice', 19.

42. 'Memorial of James Russell Clin. Prof[r] of Surgery in the University of Edinburgh to the Right Hon[ble] Charles Yorke . . . in favour of appointment Mr John Thomson his colleague in office', PRO HO 102/19 fo. 7.

43. Thomson, 'Biographical notice', 21–2.
44. Francis Horner to John Thomson, 10 January 1804, LSE R(SR) 1054, vol. 2, fo. 72.
45. Thomson, 'Biographical notice', 22.
46. 'Lectures on military surgery, by John Thomson, one of the surgeons to the Royal Infirmary', GUL MS 1476, Box 24.
47. Thomson, 'Biographical notice', 27.
48. J. Thomson to Andrew Wood and Benjamin Bell, [1804], GUL MS 1476, Box 24.
49. 'Memorial to the Royal College of Surgeons', ibid,
50. RCSE Minutes, 1793–1810, 530–1.
51. Ibid., 531–2.
52. Ibid., 533–4.
53. Ibid., 534–5.
54. EUL MS, College Minutes, 1790–1811, vol. 2, 330.
55. ECA, Council Records, 1804–5, vol. 141, 78–9.
56. J. Thomson, *Additional Hints Respecting the Improvement of the System of Medical Instruction followed in the University of Edinburgh; Humbly submitted to the Consideration of the Patrons and Professors of that Institution* (Edinburgh, 1826), 22.
57. ECA, Council Records, 1804–5, vol. 141, 98.
58. C. Hope to W. Dundas, 20 November 1804, PRO HO 102/19, fo. 174.
59. GUL MS 1476, Box 24.
60. J. Thomson to [Army Medical Board], [November? 1804], ibid.
61. 'Minutes of Army Medical Board', PRO WO 30/84.
62. 'Extracts from the Records of the Royal College of Surgeons respecting the appointment of a professorship of Surgery &c'., GUL MS 1476, Box 24.
63. [Notes on the professorship of surgery at the Royal College of Surgeons c. 1805], GUL MS 1476, Box 24, [8–9].
64. EUL MS, College Minutes, 1790–1811, vol. 2, 336–8, 369.
65. Ibid., 242–3.
66. PRO HO 102/19, fo. 7.
67. Thomson, 'Biographical notice', 29–30.
68. H. Cockburn, *Memorials of His Time* (Edinburgh, 1856), 214; Holland, *Memoirs*, 230.
69. Horner to D. Stewart, 8 February 1806, LSE R(SR) 1054, vol. 3, fo. 17.
70. *Evidence, Oral and Documentary, Taken and Received by the Commissioners Appointed . . . for Visiting the Universities of Scotland* (London, 1837), vol. 2, 205–6.
71. D. Stewart to J. Thomson, 20 February 1806, BL Additional MS 38746, fo. 227.
72. J. Bell, *Memorial Concerning the Present State of Military and Naval Surgery. Addressed to the Honourable Earl Spencer, First Lord of the Admiralty; and Now Submitted to the Public* (Edinburgh, 1800), 8.
73. Ibid., 14.
74. Ibid., 26–8.
75. PRO HO 120/19, fo. 323.
76. F. Horner to J.A. Murray, 23 January 1806, LSE R(SR) 1054, vol. 3, fo. 7.
77. EUL, College Minutes, 1790–1811, vol. 2, 396.
78. PRO WO 7/107, fo. 211.
79. J. Thomson to M. Thomson, 12 July 1815, NLS MS 9236 fo. 57.
80. J. Thomson to M. Thomson, 19 July 1815, ibid. fo. 63.
81. Thomson, 'Biographical notice', 46–8. See also: J. Thomson *Observations on the Treatment of Syphilis without Mercury* (Edinburgh, 1817), 4.

82. Anon. to William Merry, 2 February 1817, BL Additional MS 48,431, fo. 51.
83. Ibid., fo. 53.
84. [J. Thomson], *Hints Respecting the Improvement of the Literary and Scientific Education of Candidates for the Degree of Doctor of Medicine in the University of Edinburgh: Humbly Submitted to the Consideration of the Patrons and Professors of that Institution; by a Graduate of King's College, Aberdeen* (Edinburgh, 1824), 21.
85. D. Hay to Melville, 16 March 1825, WIHM MS 5122/116–123.
86. *Evidence*, vol. 1, 291.
87. Bell, *Memorial*, 23.
88. Thomson, 'Biographical notice', 42–3.
89. Ibid., 32–3.
90. GUL MS Gen. 1476, Box 24.
91. A. Monro to R. Saunders Dundas, 16 September 1808, WIHM MS 5122/1–31.
92. [W. Thomson], 'Notice of the leading events in the life of the late Dr John Thomson', *Edinburgh Medical and Surgical Journal*, (1847), 177. This passage does not appear in the later version of this biography.
93. J.B. Morrell, 'Science and Scottish university reform: Edinburgh in 1826', *British Journal for the History of Science* (1972), 44.
94. H. Monteith to Melville, 18 December 1819, WIHM MS 5122/1–3.
95. R. Graham to Melville, 21 December 1819 WIHM MS; J. Drummond to Melville, 23 December 1819, WIHM MS 5122.
96. *The Scotsman*, no. 155, 13.
97. On the contest for the practice of medicine chair see Lawrence, 'The Edinburgh medical school', 273.
98. J. Thomson, *Testimonials Presented to the Right Hon. the Lord Provost, the Magistrates, and Town Council of Edinburgh* (Edinburgh, 1821).
99. NLS MS 19339, fo. 3.
100. G. Birkbeck to J. Allen, 2 May 1821, BL Additional MS 52194, fo. 179.
101. Lauderdale to John Allen, [17-26 April 1821], BL Additional MS 52180, fo. 140.
102. Duke of York to Lord Provost of Edinburgh, 29 May 1821, WIHM MS 5122/32–63.
103. *The Scotsman*, no. 227, 167.
104. *The Scotsman*, no. 229, 181.
105. Ibid.
106. *The Scotsman*, no. 238, 255.
107. On the background to the establishment of the Commission see Morrell, 'Science and Scottish university reform', 40–1.
108. Thomson, *Hints*, 19–20.
109. Ibid., 14.
110. Ibid., 15.
111. J. Thomson, *Additional Hints* (Edinburgh, 1826), 45–6, 50.
112. Ibid., 57–8.
113. Ibid., 56.
114. Ibid., 58–9.
115. *Evidence*, vol. 1, 465–70.
116. W.P. Alison, J.H. Bennett and R. Christison, *Observations on the System of Clinical Instruction in the Royal Infirmary of Edinburgh* (Edinburgh, 1848), 6.
117. Thomson, *Additional Hints*, 64.
118. J. Thomson to J. Allen, 14 March [1827], BL Additional MS 52195, fo. 175.
119. A fact which the *Lancet* did not fail to note. It claimed that 'four successive

chairs have been created by and for Dr JOHN THOMSON, with the aid of his able political associate and Whig friend, the private secretary of Holland House!' *Lancet* (1833–4) 2, 167.

120. Lansdowne to J. Allen, 30 October [1827], ibid., fo. 208.
121. M. Napier to J. Allen, 23 April 1831, BL Additional MS 52182, fo. 135.
122. Napier to J. Allen, 13 May 1831, ibid., fo. 135.
123. F. Jeffrey to G. Lamb, 11 September 1831, SRO HH5/6. For the text of Thomson's application to the crown see W. Thomson, *Letter to the Fellows of the Royal College of Surgeons of Edinburgh, Respecting the Proposal to Abolish the Chair of General Pathology in the University* (Edinburgh, 1837), 3–5.
124. SRO HH5/6. Dated 14 September 1831.
125. EUL, College Minutes, 28 September 1831, vol. 5, 1829–37, 89–90.
126. Ibid., 91–4.
127. Ibid., 94–5.
128. ECA, Council Reports, vol. 210, 370–3.
129. J. Thomson, *Copy of a LETTER to George Aitchison, Esq. College Baillie, containing some Remarks on a Communication from the Senatus Academicus to the Patrons of the University of Edinburgh* (Edinburgh, 1831), 6.
130. Ibid., 32.
131. F. Jeffrey to G. Lamb, 26 October 1831, PRO HO 102/41, fo. 174.
132. ECA, Council Reports, vol. 211, 71–2.
133. Ibid., vol. 214, 346–8.
134. J. Duns, *Memoir of Sir James Y. Simpson, Bart.* (Edinburgh, 1873), 37–8.
135. ECA, Council Reports, vol. 213, 315.
136. Indeed in 1834 a commentator remarked that 'It would not surprise the writer to hear of an application to the patrons to allow [Thomson's] son to lecture for him – of course, without any view of subsequently slipping him in as successor' (Anon., *An Examination into the Causes of the Declining Reputation of the Medical Faculty of the University of Edinburgh; and the Origin of Another Class of Medical Professors, commonly called 'Private Lecturers;' With some Remarks on the History of the University of Edinburgh* (Edinburgh, 1834), 7).
137. ECA, Council Reports, vol. 222, 102–3.
138. Duns, *Memoir*, 82.
139. 'Memorial to Lord John Russell from Lord Provost and Town Council of Edinburgh', ECA, Council Reports, vol. 224, inserted at 372; 3–4.
140. Ibid., 5.
141. *The Scotsman*, 12 July 1837.
142. W. Thomson to J. Allen, 10 August 1837, NLS MS 9710, fo. 131.
143. J. Allen to Lord John Russell, [13 August 1837], ibid., fo. 129.
144. J. Allen to M. Napier, [30 October 1837], BL Additional MS 34618, fo. 317.
145. *The Scotsman*, 5 July 1837.
146. R. Knox, *Letter to the Right Honourable the Lord Provost and Town-Council of Edinburgh* (Edinburgh, 1837), 6.
147. R. Knox, *Second Letter to the Right Honourable the Lord Provost and Town-Council of Edinburgh* (Edinburgh, 1837), 2.
148. Anon. *An Examination*, 7.
149. Russell to J. Spittal, 16 October 1837, PRO HO 103/8, fo. 211.
150. ECA, Council Reports, vol. 228, 189.
151. Ibid., 268.
152. Thomson, *Copy*, 11–12.
153. Thomson, *An Account*, vol. 1, 500–4.
154. Ibid., vol. 1, 109.

155. Ibid., 153.
156. Ibid., 161.
157. J. Allen to E. Ellice, 27 August 1840, NLS MS 15002, fo. 23.

4 Pathologists and practitioners

1. A. Duncan, 'Lectures on the theory of medicine' (1797), EUL MS Dc. 3. 96., 7.
2. C. Bell to J. Allen, 1 December [1835], BL Additional MS 52197 fo. 20.
3. J. Thomson, *Lectures on Inflammation, Exhibiting a View of the General Doctrines, Pathological and Practical, of Medical Surgery* (Edinburgh, 1813).
4. See E. Milligan to J. Thomson, 12 November 1827, GUL MS Gen. 1476, Box 24. When he visited Edinburgh in 1826 John James Audobon made Thomson's house one of his first calls: M.R. Audobon, *Audobon and his Journals* (2 vols, London, 1898), vol. 1, 147, 153–5.
5. W. Thomson, 'Biographical notice of Dr Thomson', reproduced with amendments in J. Thomson, *An Account of the Life, Lectures, and Writings of William Cullen, M.D.* (2 vols, Edinburgh, 1859), vol. 1, 27.
6. J. Thomson, *Testimonials Presented to the Right Hon. the Lord Provost, the Magistrates, and Town Council of Edinburgh* (Edinburgh, 1821), 7.
7. Thomson, 'Biographical notice', 19–21, 25–6.
8. Thomson, *Testimonials*, 13.
9. M. Barfoot, 'Pedagogy, practice and politics: the Edinburgh medical community in the 18th century', unpublished paper.
10. Thomson, 'Biographical notice', 32–3.
11. 'Dr Thomson's Introd. Lect. Surgery', (w/m 1818/9), GUL MS Gen. 1476, Box 24, 60–1.
12. J. Bell, *Letters on Professional Character and Manners: On the Education of a Surgeon, and the Duties and Qualifications of a Physician: Addressed to James Gregory, M.D.* (Edinburgh, 1810), 548–9.
13. GUL MS Gen. 1476, Box 7 (10) (w/m 1816).
14. 'Notes of John Thomson's surgical lectures at the Royal College of Surgeons of Edinburgh', 1809, RCPE M.5. 35–6, vol. 1, 5–6.
15. Ibid., 6.
16. 'Lectures on military surgery, by John Thomson', GUL MS Gen. 1476, Box 24.
17. Thomson, *Lectures on Inflammation*, 1–2.
18. Thomson, *An Account*, vol. 1, 488.
19. 'Dr Thomson's Introd. Lect. Surgery', 2–4.
20. R.C. Maulitz, *Morbid Appearances: The Anatomy of Pathology in the Early Nineteenth Century* (Cambridge, 1987), Part 1.
21. ['Notes on proximate causes'] (w/m 1810/1816), GUL MS Gen. 1476, Box 24, 2–3.
22. Ibid., 3–4.
23. Ibid., 5.
24. O. Temkin, 'The role of surgery in the rise of modern medical thought', *Bulletin of the History of Medicine* (1951), 248–59.
25. 'Notes on proximate causes', 5–6.
26. Ibid., 9–10.
27. See D. Craigie, *Elements of General and Pathological Anatomy, Adapted to the Present State of Knowledge in that Science* (Edinburgh, 1828), viii.

28. Thomson, 'Biographical notice', 55–6.
29. 'Notes on proximate causes', 7–8.
30. 'Introductory lectures on surgery', (w/m 1810), GUL MS Gen. 1476, Box 24, 7–8.
31. ['Notes on diseases of the urinary tract'] (w/m 1810), GUL MS 1476, Box 24, [10–11].
32. Ibid., 12–13.
33. Ibid., 13–15.
34. Ibid., 17, 32–3. Thomson had in 1800 noted the claim of some French chemists to have performed successful experiments to dissolve calculi: A.F. Fourcroy, *Elements of Chemistry and Natural History. To which is prefixed, the Philosophy of Chemistry. With Notes, by John Thomson, Surgeon, Edinburgh*, 5th edn (3 vols, Edinburgh, 1800), vol. 1, 333.
35. J.B. Morrell, 'Practical chemistry in the University of Edinburgh, 1799–1843', *Ambix* (1969), 66–80; Christopher Lawrence, 'Alexander Monro *primus* and the Edinburgh manner of anatomy', *Bulletin of the History of Medicine* (1988), 193–214. For the general use of spectacle in eighteenth-century natural philosophy see S. Schaffer, 'Natural philosophy and public spectacle in the eighteenth century', *History of Science* (1983), 1–43.
36. Thomson, 'Biographical notice', 28.
37. J. Beer, *Lehre von der Augenkrankheiten* (2 vols, Wien, 1792); A.P. Demours, *Traité des Maladies des Yeux* (4 vols, Paris, 1818); W. Adams, *Practical Observations on Ectropium, or Eversion of the Eye-lids* (London, 1812); J. Wardrop, *Essays on the Morbid Anatomy of the Human Eye*, (2 vols, Edinburgh, 1808–18).
38. *Biographical sketch of the late John Alexander Schetky*, EUL Pamphlet Q.P. 123/19, 2.
39. Thomson, 'Biographical sketch', 56.
40. J. Abernethy, *Surgical Observations, Containing a Classification of Tumours* (London, 1804).
41. Dr Thomson's Lect. Surgery, 26.
42. J. Wardrop, *Observations on Fungus Haematodes or Soft Cancer, in Several of the most Important Organs of the Human Body: Containing also a Comparative View of the Structure of Fungus Haematodes and Cancer. With Cases and Dissections* (Edinburgh, 1809).
43. Cf. M. Foucault, *The Birth of the Clinic: An Archaeology of Medical Perception* (London, 1989), 88–9.
44. ['Lecture on anatomy',] (w/m 1816), GUL MS Gen. 2251, Box 7 [10].
45. 'Diseases of subcutaneous cellular tissue', GUL MS Gen. 1476, Box 4, [14, 21].
46. Maulitz, *Morbid Appearances*, esp. 143–5.
47. 'Dr Thomson's Introd. Lect. Surgery', 44.
48. Thomson, 'Biographical notice', 43.
49. Thomson, *Testimonials*, 29–30.
50. J. Thomson to M. Thomson, 18 November 1814, NLS MS 9236 fo. 43.
51. Thomson, 'Biographical notice', 50.
52. J. Thomson, ['Journal'], NLS MS 9235, 22.
53. J. Thomson to M. Thomson, 13 August 1814, NLS MS 9236 fo. 28.
54. Thomson, 'Journal', 23.
55. J. Thomson to M. Thomson, 13 August 1814.
56. Thomson had expressed a special wish to meet Cuvier: 'As Dr Thomson's studies have a very close affinity to some favourite pursuits of Mr Cuvier, he is anxious to be known to that Gentleman' (D. Stewart to [Joseph Marie] de Gérando, 17 July 1814, NLS MS 5319, fo. 48).

57. Thomson, 'Journal', 25–6.
58. Ibid., 37.
59. J. Thomson to M. Thomson, 13 August 1814.
60. Ibid., 21.
61. Ibid., 38–9.
62. J. Thomson to M. Thomson, 13 August 1814.
63. J. Thomson to M. Thomson, 5 September 1814, NLS MS 9236 fo. 36.
64. Thomson, 'Journal', 31, 33–4.
65. Ibid., 35–7.
66. Ibid., 38.
67. See S.J. Reiser, *Medicine and the Reign of Technology* (Cambridge, 1978), ch. 2.
68. 'Notes of medical cases made in France 1822–5', EUL MS Gen. 590, 132.
69. Thomson, 'Biographical notice', 62–3.
70. Laennec died in 1826.
71. ['Lectures on Institutes of Medicine'], GUL MS Gen. 1476, Box 25; 'Respiration', 331–2.
72. 'Pathology by Dr Thomson of the Edinburgh University' (1837), EUL MS Dc. 3. 110, 79, 77.
73. Ibid., 104.
74. Hodgkin MSS, Friends House London, Microfilm 480.
75. I have discussed this more fully in 'Robert Carswell and William Thomson at the Hôtel-Dieu of Lyons: Scottish views of French medicine', in R. French and A. Wear (eds), *British Medicine in an Age of Reform* (London, 1991), 110–33.
76. John Thomson to William Clift, 21 May 1822, BL Additional MS 39954, vol. 1, fo. 3.
77. J. Thomson to W. Thomson, 4 July 1822, NLS MS 9236 fo. 111.
78. Ibid.
79. Ibid.
80. J. Thomson to W. Thomson, ibid., fo. 123.
81. See B. Latour, *Science in Action: How to Follow Scientists and Engineers through Society* (Milton Keynes, 1987), 224–5.
82. Henry Halford to Allen, 18 December 1822, BL Additional MS 52195, fo. 37.
83. Allen to Halford, 19 December 1822, ibid., fo. 39.
84. Ibid.
85. Thomson, 'Biographical notice', 57.
86. Anon. *An Examination into the Causes of the Declining Reputation of the Medical Faculty of the University of Edinburgh; And the Origin of Another Class of Medical Professors, Commonly called 'Private Lecturers;' With some Remarks on the History of the University of Edinburgh* (Edinburgh, 1834).
87. W.P. Alison, *Letter to the Right Honourable the Lord Provost, Magistrates, and Town-Council of Edinburgh, in Explanation of the Proposal of the Professors Relative to the Chair of General Pathology* (Edinburgh, 1837), 9.
88. J. Syme, *Letter to the Right Hon. the Lord Provost, Magistrates, and Town-Council of Edinburgh* (Edinburgh, 1837), 6-7.
89. Maulitz, *Morbid Appearances*, 216–18.
90. Quoted ibid., 218.
91. Carswell to John Thomson, 5 July 1831, GUL MS Gen. 1476, Box 24.
92. GUL MS Gen. 1476, Box 18.
93. The collection was eventually purchased by the University of Edinburgh in 1857 due to the efforts of the then Professor of the Practice of Medicine, Thomas Laycock. See EUL, College Minutes, 1855–61, 135, 140, 148.

94. Charles J.B. Williams, *Memoirs of Life and Works* (London 1884), 17–18. Williams also noted that Thomson's lectures were of less use as an introduction to the practice of medicine.

95. ['Lectures on institutes of medicine'], 'Lecture I', GUL MS Gen. 1476, Box 25, 65.

96. Thomson, 'Biographical notice', 86.

97. 'Lecture I', 17–8.

98. Ibid., 15.

99. See M.S. Staum, 'Cabanis and the revolution: The therapy of society', in H. Woolf (ed.), *The Analytic Spirit* (Ithaca, 1981), 146–74; idem, *Cabanis: Enlightenment and Medical Philosophy in the French Revolution* (Princeton, 1980); L.S. Jacyna, 'Medical science and moral science: The cultural relations of physiology in restoration France', *History of Science* (1987), 111–46.

100. Quoted in J. Thomson, *Hints Respecting the Improvement of the Literary and Scientific Education of Candidates for the Degree of Doctor of Medicine in the University of Edinburgh: Humbly Submitted to the Consideration of the Patrons and Professors of that Institution; by a Graduate of King's College, Aberdeen* (Edinburgh, 1824), 6–7.

101. 'Lectures on mental faculties and nervous system', GUL MS Gen. 1476, Box 25, 1. Thomson had a long-standing interest in mental disease. During his time in Paris he visited the insane housed in the Salpêtrière noting that: 'I walk through the streets of the madhouse in all states without seeing any of the disagreeable sensations I would have had in my own Country – I believe this is owing to my ignorance of the French language – what they say does not affect me' (Thomson, 'Journal', 33).

102. Ibid., 5–6.

103. Ibid., 11–12.

104. Ibid., 57–8.

105. 'Lectures on the institutes of medicine', Lecture V, 24–8. T. Reid, *Essays on the powers of the human mind* (3 vols, Edinburgh, 1803).

106. D. Stewart, *Elements of the Philosophy of the Human Mind* (3 vols, London and Edinburgh, 1792, 1814, 1827).

107. 'Mental faculties and nervous system', Lecture I, 48–9.

108. 'Lectures on institutes of medicine', Lecture V, 2.

109. Ibid., 16.

110. See B. Hoppe, 'Le concepte de biologie chez G.R. Treviranus', *Colloque International 'Lamarck'* (Paris, 1971); L.J. Jordanova, *Lamarck* (Oxford, 1984), esp. ch. 5; P. Corsi, *The Age of Lamarck: Evolutionary Theories in France 1790–1830* (Berkeley, 1988).

111. [Fragment dated 29 June 1827], GUL MS Gen. 1476, Box 3.

112. [Fragment] (w/m 1819), ibid.

113. 'Lectures on institutes of medicine', V, 48–9.

114. 'General account of the vegetable kingdom. Vegetable physiology', GUL MS Gen. 1476, Box 3.

115. 'Animal functions those of mind & body – of locomotion sensation & consciousness – or sensation consciousness & volition', GUL MS Gen. 1476, Box 3.

116. 'Blood and circulation', GUL MS Gen. 1476, Box 25, 19–24.

117. A. Desmond, 'Robert E. Grant: the social predicament of a pre-Darwinian transmutationist', *Journal of the History of Biology* (1984), 200–2.

118. See P. Corsi, 'The importance of French transformist ideas for the second volume of Lyell's Principles of Geology', *British Journal for the History of Science* (1978), 221–44.

119. Jordanova, *Lamarck*, 78.
120. A. Desmond, 'Artisan resistance and evolution in Britain, 1819–1848', *Osiris* (1987), 77–110.
121. Thomson, 'Biographical notice', 82.
122. [Fragment] (w/m 182–), GUL MS Gen. 1476, Box 3.
123. Compare W.P. Alison, *Outlines of Physiology: With an Appendix, containing Heads of Lectures on Pathology and Therapeutics* (Edinburgh, 1831), 2.
124. Knox made no bones of his hostility to Thomson see R. Knox, *Second Letter to the Right Honourable the Lord Provost and Town-Council of Edinburgh* (Edinburgh, 1837), esp. 7.
125. In December 1825, for instance, Thomson had 204 appointments: GUL MS Gen. 1476, Box 18.
126. 'Mr Scott's case', GUL MS Gen. 1476, Box 18, 15.
127. Ibid., 1.
128. J. Robertson to Thomson, 19 October 1829, GUL MS Gen. 1476, Box 18.
129. R. Liston to Thomson, 29 July 1834, NLS 4039 fo. 77; Thomson to Liston, ibid., fo. 322A.
130. J. Tod to J. Thomson, 5 November 1827; J. Cunningham to Thomson, 1827; T. Dallas to Thomson, 5 December 1827; J.M. Threipland to Thomson, 25 March 1827; Nimmo to Thomson, 16 October 1827: all in GUL MS Gen. 1476, Box 18.
131. Thomson, 'Biographical notice', 48. W. Jamieson to Thomson, 16 September 1834, GUL MS Gen. 1476, Box 18.
132. Ibid., 63–4.
133. [Notes on wound healing] (w/m 1816/1818), GUL MS Gen. 1476, Box 24, 7–8.
134. 'Syphilis cured without mercury', *Edinburgh Medical and Surgical Journal* (1817), 250–1.
135. Thomson, 'Biographical notice', 78–9.
136. Ibid., 79.
137. A. Coats to Thomson, 26 November 1833, GUL MS Gen. 1476, Box 18.
138. M. Thomson to W. Thomson, [1822], NLS MS 9236 fo. 125.
139. Ibid.
140. Anon. to W. Merry, 2 February 1817, BL Additional MS 48431 fo. 50.
141. Thomson to Allen, 10 June 1828, NLS MS 583 fo. 720.
142. C. Findlater to Thomson, 2 and 19 July 1832, GUL MS Gen. 1476, Box 18.
143. N.D. Jewson, 'Medical knowledge and the patronage system in eighteenth-century England', *Sociology* (1974), 369–85; idem, 'The disappearance of the sick man from medical cosmology', *Sociology* (1976), 225–44.
144. 'From my little acquaintance with anatomy I know not how far or in what direction sympathy of parts (if the shade of Dr Cullen does not rise to protest against the phrase) does act. I have often been affected with *lumbago* – but think that since my other complaint, it is more constant tho' not at all severe or acute' (Findlater to Thomson, 19 July 1832).
145. Thomson divided mankind into five 'temperaments': sanguineous, leucophlegmatic, atrabilious or melancholic, bilious, and nervous. He added that the last was 'an important addition of modern times'. These constitutional differences 'have a great power in modifying the symptoms and producing different kinds of disease' ('Pathology by Dr Thomson', 19).
146. See G. Risse, 'Doctor William Cullen, physician, Edinburgh: a consultation practice in the eighteenth century', *Bulletin of the History of Medicine* (1974), 338–51.
147. G. White to Thomson, 29 December 1829, GUL MS Gen. 1476, Box 18.
148. W. Carnegy [?] to Thomson, 13 October 1831, GUL MS Gen. 1476, Box 18.

149. R. Moir to Thomson, 5 April 1828, ibid. A number of records of autopsies undertaken in the course of Thomson's practice are preserved: see EUL MS Gen. 591, 95–9.
150. G. Kelly to Thomson, undated, EUL MS Gen. 591, 75–6.
151. White to Thomson, 20 February 1830, ibid.
152. J. Armstrong to Thomson, 24 February 1828, ibid.
153. J. Stenhouse to Thomson, 27 December 1821, ibid., 77.
154. C. Cheyne to Thomson, 11 September 1827, ibid., 83–4.
155. See A. Jamieson to Thomson, 8 July 1822, ibid., 87–8.

5 A Whig decline

1. These details are taken from A. Thomson, 'Biographical notice of Dr William Thomson', in J. Thomson, *An Account of the Life, Lectures, and Writings of William Cullen, M.D.* (2 vols, Edinburgh, 1859), vol. 1, 85–92.
2. A note of these lectures dated 7 December 1822 is in the Cullen Papers, GUL MS Gen. 2225, Box 6.
3. Ibid., Box 1, 16. Although I have ascribed these manuscripts to William Thomson, they appear to be the result of collective notetaking by him and his companions that was later compiled into a single document.
4. Ibid., 22.
5. Ibid., 23.
6. Ibid., 28.
7. Ibid., 30.
8. Ibid., 35.
9. W. Thomson, *A Probationary Essay in the Extraction of Calculi from the Urinary Bladder, containing some Account of certain Methods that have been proposed, submitted by Authority of the President and Council, to the Examination of the Royal College of Surgeons of Edinburgh, when a Candidate for Admission into their Body, in Conformity to their Regulations respecting the Admission of Ordinary Fellows* (Edinburgh, 1825).
10. J. Thomson to J. Allen, 14 March [1827], BL Additional MS 52195 fo. 175.
11. W. Thomson to Andrew, Lord Rutherfurd, 21 August 1840, NLS MS 9712 fo. 22.
12. On Rutherfurd see G.W.T. Osmond, *The Lord Advocates of Scotland: Second Series 1834–1880* (London, 1914), 47–125.
13. Thomson to Rutherfurd, 21 August 1840.
14. Ibid., fo. 24, adapted.
15. W. Thomson to J. Oswald, 28 August 1840, NLS MS 9712 fo. 30.
16. SRO HH 5/16.
17. *Evidence, Oral and Documentary, Taken and Received by the Commissioners Appointed . . . for visiting the Universities of Scotland* (London, 1837), vol. 2, 214.
18. Ibid., 137.
19. W. Thomson to Andrew, Lord Rutherfurd, 14 November 1848, NLS MS 9714 ffo. 300–301.
20. 'Minutes of the Plinian Society', EUL MS Dc. 2. 53, vol. 1, 68.
21. See L.S. Jacyna, '*Au lit des malades*: A.F. Chomel's clinic at the Charité, 1828–9', *Medical History* (1989), 420–49.
22. Thomson's situation as a practitioner dealing with aristocratic patients in many respects resembled that outlined in N. Jewson, 'Medical knowledge and the patronage system in eighteenth-century England', *Sociology* (1974), 369–85.
23. Allen Thomson to J. Thomson, 28 June 1836, NLS MS 9237 fo. 6.
24. Allen Thomson to J. Thomson, 23 October [1836], ibid., fo. 15.

25. Ibid.
26. Allen Thomson to Margaret Thomson junior, 9 July 1837, ibid., fo. 77.
27. Ibid., fo. 15.
28. Allen Thomson to Margaret Thomson senior, [1836], ibid., fo. 100.
29. Allen Thomson to J. Thomson, 23 October 1836.
30. Allen Thomson to Margaret Thomson senior, 1836.
31. Allen Thomson to J. Thomson, 23 October 1836.
32. Ibid.
33. Ibid.
34. Allen Thomson to J. Thomson, 24 February [1837], ibid., fo. 43.
35. 'Minutes of the Plinian Society', vol. 1, 74–5.
36. Ibid.
37. Ibid.
38. See J.R. Poynter, *Society and Pauperism: English Ideas on Poor Relief, 1795-1834* (London, 1969), 234–7. Contrast the ideas on poverty of another Edinburgh physician, William Pulteney Alison: R.A. Cage, *The Scottish Poor Law 1745-1845* (Edinburgh, 1981), 125–30.
39. Allen Thomson to John Thomson, 24 February 1837. The applicability of a system of relief to Irish society had agitated commentators since the 1820s. See Poynter, *Society*, 306–10.
40. Allen Thomson to J. Thomson, 30 July [1836], NLS MS 9237, fo. 79. See also: L.S. Jacyna (ed.), *A Tale of Three Cities: The Correspondence of William Sharpey and Allen Thomson* (London, 1989), 1–5.
41. Allen Thomson to J. Thomson, 1 June [1837], ibid., fo. 62; A. Thomson to M. Thomson, 9 July [1837].
42. Allen Thomson to Margaret Thomson senior, [1837], ibid. fo. 82.
43. Allen Thomson to Margaret Thomson senior, 26 March [1836], ibid. fo. 55.
44. Allen Thomson to J. Thomson, 23 October 1836.
45. Allen Thomson to Margaret Thomson junior, [1836], NLS 9237 fo. 33.
46. Alen Thomson to J. Thomson, 5 June [1837], ibid., fo. 68.
47. Ibid.
48. M. Thomson senior to Allen Thomson, 8 June 1837, ibid., fo. 74.
49. W. Aitken, ['Obituary of Allen Thomson'], *Proceedings of the Royal Society of London* (1887), xvi.
50. W. Sharpey to Allen Thomson, 25 January 1848, Jacyna, *Tale of Three Cities*, 62.
51. Ibid., 13.
52. Ibid., 16.
53. Ibid., 17–18.
54. Aitken, 'Obituary', xiv.
55. Even before this scandal feeling against dissection was reputed to be especially strong in Scotland: [William Foster], *An Answer to the Several Attacks which have appeared against the University of Edinburgh. Together with a Comparative View of the Lectures of the Late Dr Gordon of Edinburgh, – of Mr Abernethy of St. Bartholomew's Hospital, – of Mr Wilson, – and of Mr C. Bell, London* (Edinburgh, 1819), 26.
56. See R. Richardson, *Death, Dissection and the Destitute* (London, 1988), esp. ch. 5.
57. 'Study of anatomy in Edinburgh', *Lancet* (1837–8), 1, 589.
58. See Richardson, *Death*, 242.
59. 'Study of anatomy', 590.
60. Thomson was well aware of Somerville's importance to the prospects of an anatomy teacher in Edinburgh; 'I must', he told his mother, 'keep him in good humor' (Allen Thomson to Margaret Thomson senior, 29 January [1836], NLS 9237 fo. 41).

61. William Campbell to William Mackenzie, 3 March 1842, GUL MS Gen. 1476, Box 18.

62. 'D^{ft} of letter to Home Secretary requesting money to build Dead Houses in Edin^{r}. A.T'., ibid.

63. 'Letter to Sir Thos D. Lauder Chair^{m} of man. of W.K. Workhouse on Supply of Dead Bodies', ibid.

64. 'Df^{t} of regulations among lecturers in Edin^{r} for distribution of bodies', ibid.

65. In November 1841 the lecturers agreed the following schedule of prices:

An Entire Adult – £3.
– Opened – £2.
– Children 5 to 10 years – Entire – £1.10.
– Children 5 to 10 years – Opened – 15.
– Children 1 to 5 years – Entire – 15.
– Children 1 to 5 – Opened – 10.
– Children under one year – opened – 10.

(W. Campbell to A. Thomson, 19 April 1842, ibid.)

66. 'Forms of agreement of teaching with the university for the distribution of bodies', ibid.

67. 'D^{ft} of letter'.

68. Campbell to Thomson, 19 April 1842.

69. 'Number of registered pupils of pract^{l} anatomy'; 'Number of registered pupils of anatomy in books of College of Surgeons 1841', ibid.

70. William Sharpey to Allen Thomson, 9 March 1839, Jacyna, *Tale of Three cities*, 24.

71. 'Lect. 1st Introductory. Edinburgh 1838 & Aberdeen 1839', GUL MS Gen. 1476, Box 7, 25–6.

72. Ibid., 28.

73. Ibid., 1–2.

74. Ibid., 22–4.

75. Ibid., 36.

76. Ibid., 15–17.

77. Ibid., 28–9.

78. Ibid., 29–30.

79. Ibid., 34.

80. Ibid., 35.

81. 'Aberdeen 2nd Novr 1840. Introductory', ibid., 6.

82. A. Thomson to R. Owen, 6 September 1841, BL Additional MS 39954, fo. 28.

83. ECA, Council Records, vol. 237, 337, 367–9.

84. 'Introductory lecture to Institutions of Medicine. 1842–43', GUL MS Gen. 1476, Box 7, 1–2. I have discussed the changes in the remit of the institute's chair more fully in: 'Theory of Medicine, science of life' in R. Porter (ed.), *The History of Medical Education*, forthcoming.

85. 'Lectures on physiology', GUL MS Gen. 170 (vol. 2), Lecture 40, [2].

86. 'Lectures on physiology', GUL MS Gen. 170 (vol. 1), 'Introductory lecture. 1832', 10.

87. Ibid., 16.

88. ['Lectures on physiology 1831–4'], GUL MS Gen. 1476, Box 3, Lecture 2, 8–9.

89. Ibid., 10–11.

90. Ibid., 12.

91. 'Notes on Mr Wilsons lectures on moral philosophy', GUL MS Gen. 1476, Box 4.

92. 'Introductory. Institutions of Medicine. Tuesday 5th Novr 1833', GUL MS Gen. 170 (vol. 1), 38–40.

93. H. Brougham, *A Discourse of Natural Theology, showing the Nature of the Advantages of the Study* (Brussels, 1835), 44.

94. Ibid., 45.

95. C. Bell, *The Hand: Its Mechanism and Vital Endowments as evincing Design* (London, 1833), 146–7.

96. J. Fletcher, *Discourse on the Importance of the Study of Physiology as a Branch of Popular Education, Delivered at Edinburgh on the 5th, and Repeated on the 10th of March 1836* (Edinburgh, 1836), 14. On Fletcher's commitment to natural theology see R. Lewis, 'Biographical memoir of Dr Fletcher', preface to J. Fletcher, *Rudiments of Physiology* (Edinburgh, 1835–7), Part III, xix.

97. Ibid., 15–16.

98. '[Lectures on physiology, c. 1831–4]', GUL MS Gen. 1476, Box 3, Lecture 2, pp. 2, 4.

99. See O. Temkin, 'German concepts of ontogeny and history around 1800', in his *The Double Face of Janus and other Essays in the History of Medicine* (Baltimore, 1977), 373–89.

100. Allen Thomson *De Evolutione Cordis in Animalibus Vertebratis*, MD thesis, Edinburgh University 1830; idem, 'On the development of the vascular system in the foetus of vertebrated animals', *Edinburgh New Philosophical Journal* (1830), 295–327; idem, 'Contributions to the history of the structure of the human ovum and embryo before the third week after conception, with a description of some early ova', *Edinburgh Medical and Surgical Journal* (1839), 119–36.

101. 'Minutes of the Plinian Society', vol. 2, 85, 119–20.

102. Allen Thomson, 'Opening address of the British Association for the Advancement of Science, 1871 Edinburgh', *Nature* (1871), 295.

103. Fletcher, *Rudiments*, Part 1, 36, 38 fn. On the wider dissemination of transcendental doctrines in Britain see L.S. Jacyna, 'Principles of general physiology: The comparative dimension to British neuroscience in the 1830s and 1840s', *Studies in History of Biology* (1984), 47–92.

104. A. Desmond, *The Politics of Evolution: Morphology, Medicine, and Reform in Radical London* (Chicago, 1989), 58–9; H. Lonsdale, *A Sketch of the Life and Writings of Robert Knox the Anatomist* (London, 1870), 244–8. For Knox's views on the limitations of teleology see R. Knox, *Contributions to Anatomy and Physiology* (London, 1843), 21–3.

105. On Knox's eccentric politics see E. Richards, 'The "moral anatomy" of Robert Knox: the interplay between biological and social thought in Victorian scientific naturalism', *Journal of the History of Biology* (1989), 373–436.

106. Fletcher, *Rudiments*, Part 1, 16–17.

107. W. Sharpey to A. Thomson, 17 February 1877, Jacyna, *Tale of Three Cities*, 139.

108. 'Lectures on physiology', (2), '48th lect. January. 18 [1834]', 1–4.

109. 'Comparative anatomy & development of the brain, [1843]', GUL MS Gen. 1476, Box 8, p. 9.

110. Ibid., '93rd lect. March 26th [1834]', 3.

111. 'Lectures on physiology [1832–5]', '36th lect. Jany 2 1833', 3.

112. Ibid., '47 th lect.', 1–2.

113. P.M. Roget, *An Introductory Lecture on Human and Comparative Physiology. Delivered at the New Medical School in Aldersgate Street* (London, 1826), 61–2.

114. W. Sharpey to A. Thomson, 31 January 1848, Jacyna, *Tale of Three Cities*, 64.

115. By 1861 Thomson's income from the anatomy chair came to £750. J. Coutts, *A History of the University of Glasgow: From its Foundation in 1451 to 1909* (Glasgow, 1909), 520–1.
116. Sharpey to Thomson, 28 December 1847, Jacyna, *Tale of Three Cities*, 61.
117. A. Thomson to Andrew, Lord Rutherfurd, 9 February 1848, NLS MS 9714 ffo. 178–9.

Epilogue

1. '[Review of] K.F.H. Marx, *Errinerungen an England*', *British and Foreign Medical Review* (1843), 20.

Index

Institutions belong to Edinburgh, unless otherwise stated.